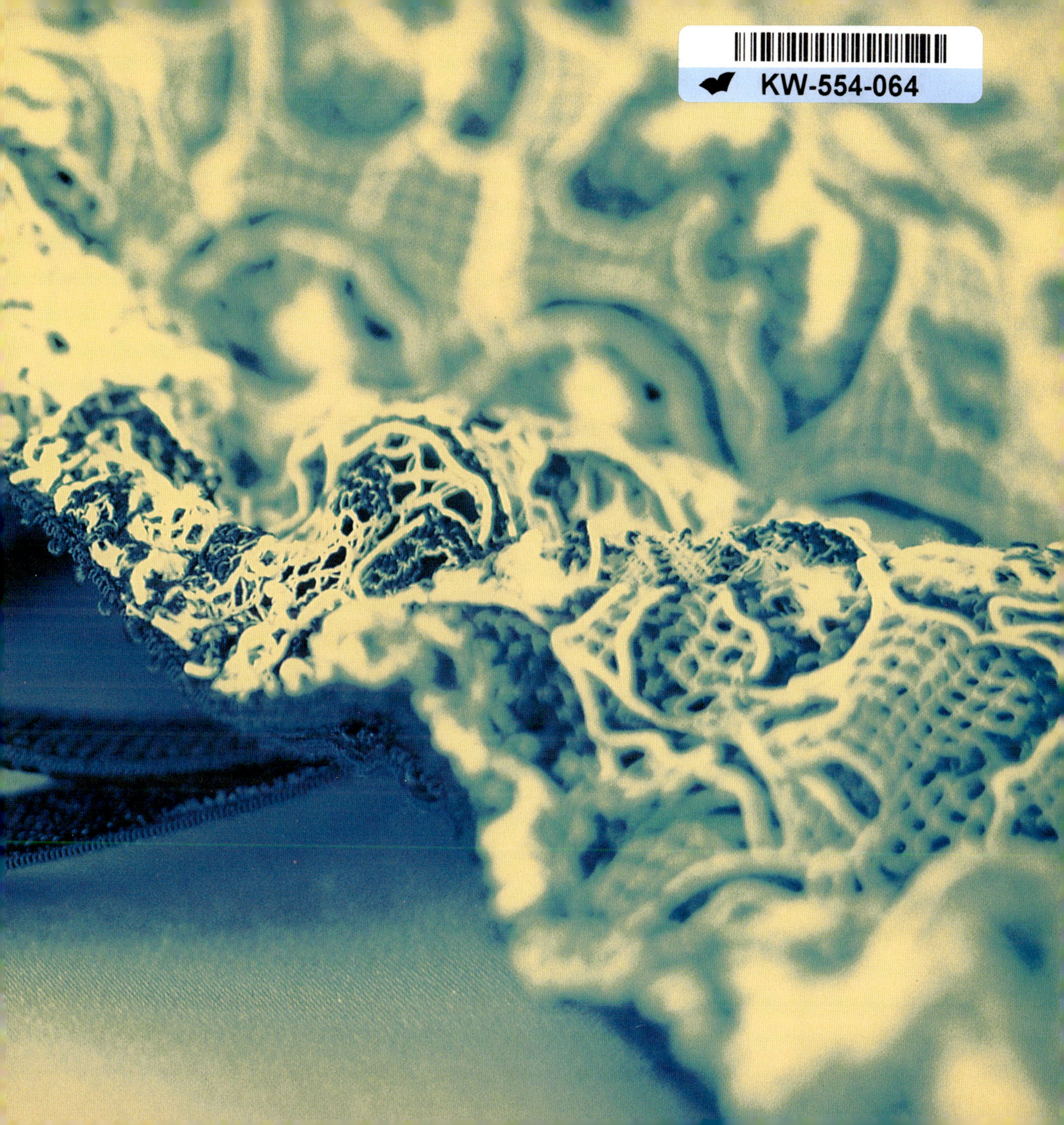

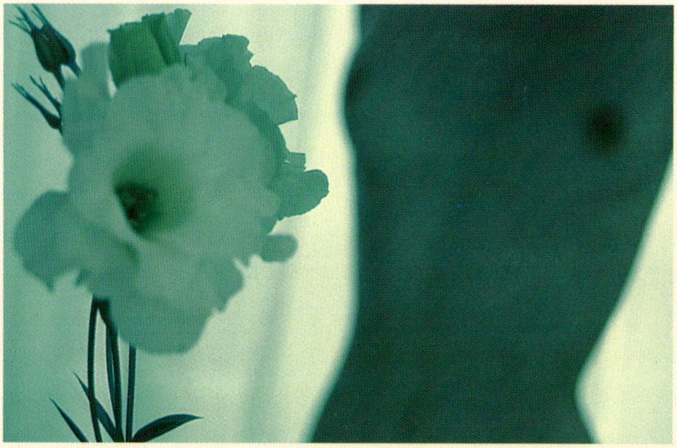

aphrodisiac

kyle cathie limited

marion mcgilvary

photographs laura hodgson

to A & A

Special thanks to Caroline and Kyle for giving us the opportunity to do this book, to Claire and Rachel for their time and advice, and to Sonya for her vision and brilliance with the graphics.

Marion would like to thank all her extremely candid friends, especially Julia, Nina, Rosie, Angie, Claire, Nancy, Sarah, Heidi, Freddie, Louise and Dima, as well as all the men she spoke to, who wish to remain nameless.

Laura would like to thank Zara, Chloë, Dan, Corina, Jeremy, Craig, Miranda, Charlotte, Benjamin, Melissa, Jason, Mark, Hannah, Chris and Alannah for modelling so beautifully; Jemima and Chris for the working holiday; and Blue, Charlie, Lucy and Camilla for all their help and support.

First published in Great Britain in 1998 by
Kyle Cathie Limited
20 Vauxhall Bridge Road
London SW1V 2SA

ISBN 1 85626 322 3

Edited by Caroline Taggart
Design by Sonya Collins at bwa design
Black and white prints by John Smith at Genesis

Marion McGilvary and Laura Hodgson are hereby identified as the authors of this work in accordance with Section 77 of the Copyright Designs and Patents Act 1988

A Cataloguing in Publication record for this title is available from the British Library.

Printed and bound in Singapore by Tien Wah Press

contents

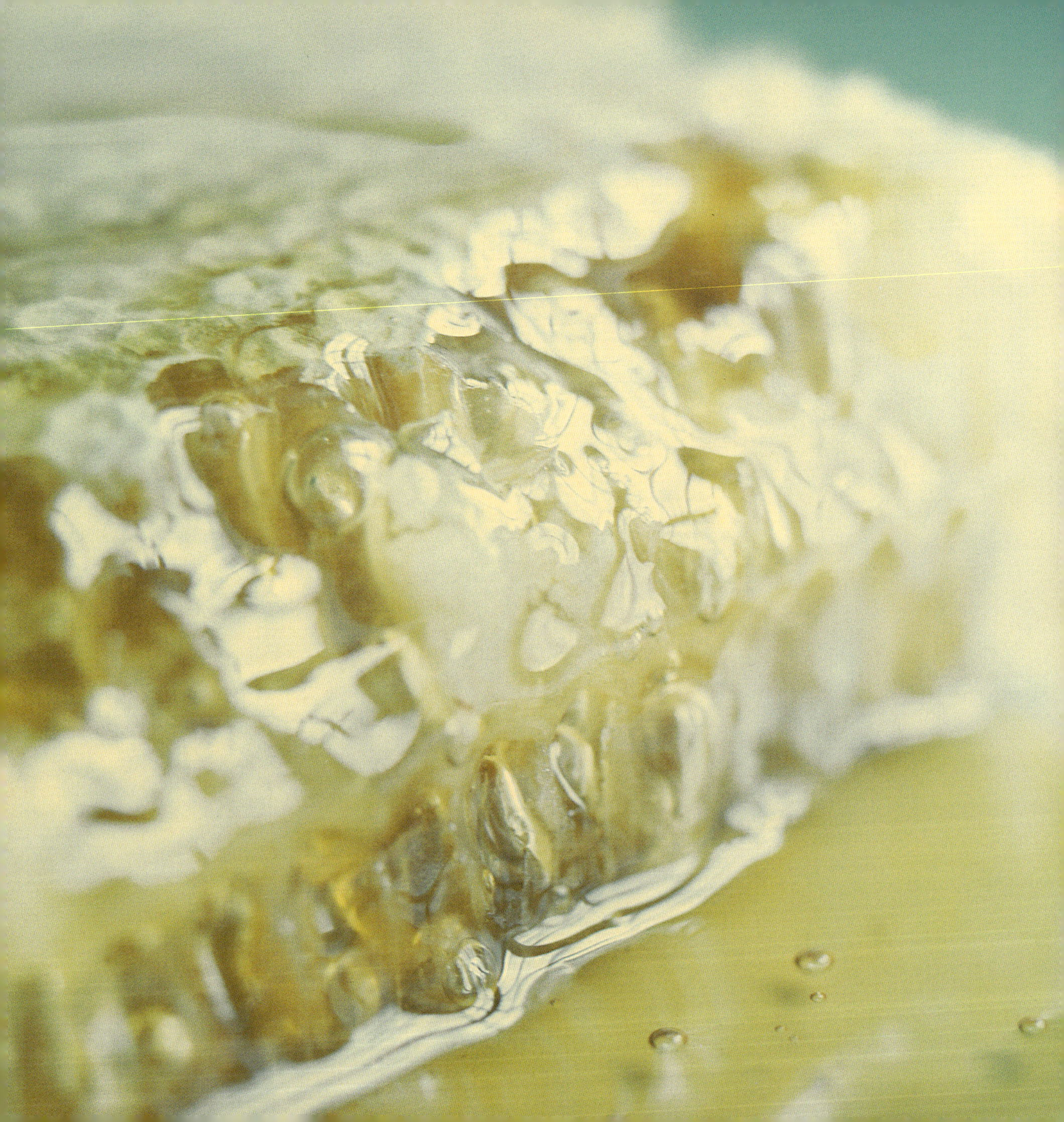

introduction

For centuries, lovers have yearned to find anything that would arouse sexual performance and enhance desire. In the search for potency, anything goes, even powdered lizard. However, as far as the modern lover is concerned, most ingredients in traditional love potions are at best impractical and at worst downright outlandish. For instance, during the Renaissance, 'goblets d'amour' contained such things as the blood of a red-haired person. Even if this did inflame your lover, it wouldn't win you many friends. Especially red-headed ones.

This book banishes such concoctions to history's basement, where they belong, and gets real. Forget carps' tongues and open a jar of caviar. Who cares what they did in classical times? Nero may have fiddled while his wife bathed in asses' milk, but most of us would prefer a flagon of something from Chanel and the fire to be burning somewhere closer to home than Rome.

By considering our responses in terms of sight, sound, touch, scent, taste and – sexiest of all – our sixth sense, *Aphrodisiac* updates the notion of what exactly constitutes sex appeal and explores contemporary ways of stimulating the libido and exhilarating your lover. So if you think the modern turn-on is something you do with a remote control and a wide-screen television, get ready to tune in to a different channel.

Aphrodisiac discusses all those things that mother nature didn't want to tell you until you were older. How to make your body into a temple and how heels, herbs and a hot bath can all help to increase the size of the congregation.

It may come as something of a shock, but you know that saying about moderation in all things? Well, it's a lie.

Women's lingerie should be worn to be seen and appreciated, but forget what your mother told you about always having a clean set of underwear on in case you get hit by a car. Dearest, if you are involved in a traffic accident the last thing you will care about is whether your silk bra and knickers match.

However, to undress for success your underwear should be glamorous. Red is what men buy for women, white is for little girls and people with nurse fantasies, and black is best. Always buy silk, never polyester or nylon – you want the atmosphere to be charged, but not with static electricity. Corsets feel like sexy strait-jackets but are fantastically effective so worth the trouble. Camisoles and French knickers are very alluring, but with lingerie, generally, the scantier the better.

The drawback with little bits of frilly lace is that they look alarmingly conspicuous when worn underneath hip-hugging clothes. Some women like thongs; others say that wearing one is akin to being garrotted by a cheese string. However, this can make you extra eager to take it off, which is surely the ultimate goal.

For those of us whose figures are like Venice – decadent, beautiful and slowly sinking into the sea – the push-up bra is the ultimate rescue remedy. But buy something frivolous, not fortified. Lingerie should be sold in little crumpled piles of froth that your fingers can dance through – and should not be bought in a supermarket. I don't care how many colour co-ordinated pairs you get in a pack. There's something so depressing about all those sad, shoddy rows of stretchy nylon satin and synthetic lace in every size from an eight to a twenty.

Women's underwear is about glamour, fantasy, promise – and the willingness to pretend that of course you always wear black satin G-string knickers to a rugby match. There's a fine line between where the sexy underwear stops and the back pages of top-shelf magazines begin. Cross it and enjoy yourself.

sight lingerie...

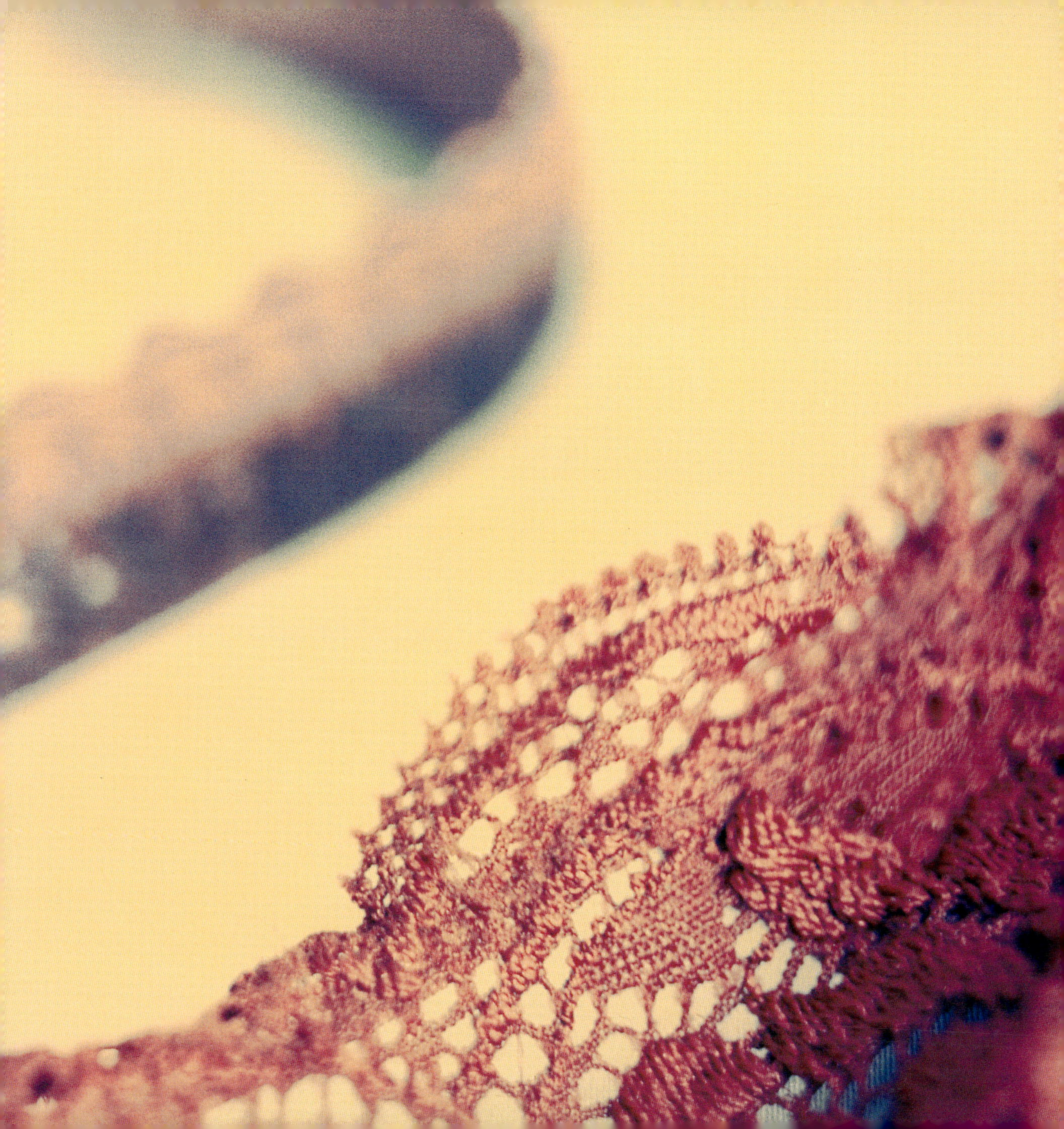

I was persuaded to like boxer shorts – and, no, I am not going to go into details. Suffice to say they pack their own punch and don't need me to defend them. Nowadays the popular choice seems to be anything with Calvin Klein stamped on the waistband.

Personally I think grown men should be way past the stage of needing to have names embroidered on their underwear, but these, or a pair of simple, well-fitted cotton trunks seem to be the best liked amongst women. Bikini briefs, according to most of my friends, are great. But only if you are either gay or Italian.

Y-fronts have made rather an unwelcome comeback into the sock drawer of life. Some young women love them – especially those in contrasting seventies colours. Well, purple pants with a pink trim round the crotch are fun – but sexy? That's a matter of opinion. I still think they should be ceremonially burnt on a specially designated day once a year when boys of an impressionable age are fast asleep. Posing pouches and thongs are fine if you have buns of steel and enough equipment to strike a pose. For buns of the softer variety, disguise them in boxers – please! Avoid anything with paisley patterns or cartoon characters. I don't care if you have had them since you were ten and have matching sheets – you are a big boy now. Aren't you...?

String underwear? She will strangle you with it, just before she runs screaming down the hallway with her knickers in her hand.

Some people seem to prefer the natural look and just leave their nether parts to air. Men find this particularly exciting in a woman, especially if told in advance – but, girls, you only have yourselves to blame when you never see the end of a film or eat dessert again.

...etc

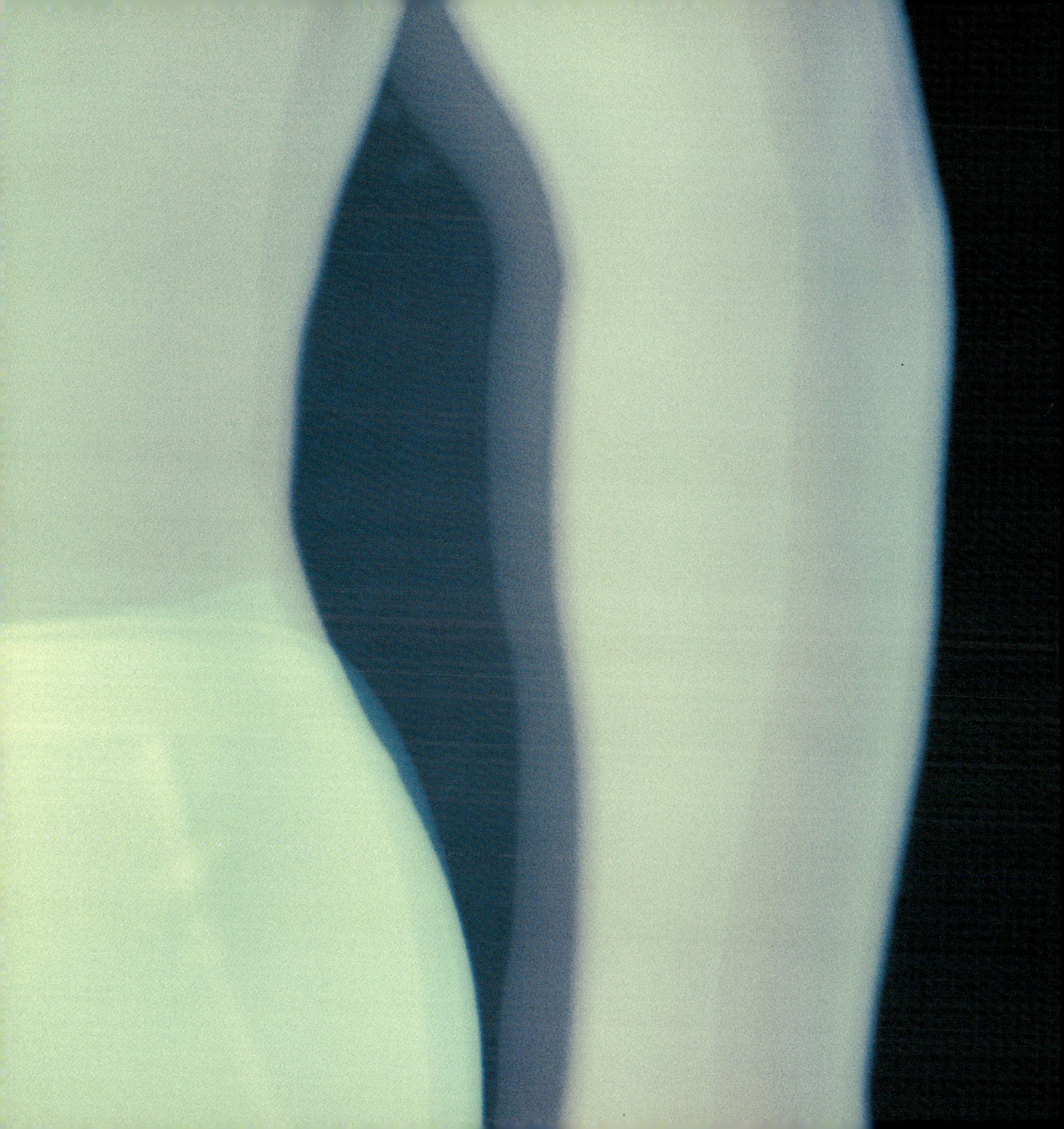

When all else fails, women buy themselves a new lipstick. I know. I have 73 identical shades of red in a variety of tubes, all of which were bought as shoe-replacement therapy.

Red lips are an overt sexual symbol. They personify glamour, sophistication and passion. It is hard to imagine any of the screen goddesses from the forties and fifties, like Marilyn Monroe or Rita Hayworth, without their bright red mouths. No sexy vamp ever swayed out into the big wide world of seduction without a bit of lippy.

It's true that glossy lipstick as seen on the covers of fashion magazines can be a turn-on, but it doesn't look quite as nice smeared across your partner's chin, ear and best Armani shirt. Modern, stay-with-you-for-life lip colours still have you red and pouting next morning, but won't leave your lover looking as if he has been branded. Be careful about choosing fashionable colours. Purple has distinct Bride-of-Frankenstein connotations, and fuchsia may be the hot new shade, but unless your partner reads the beauty section regularly he could mistake you for a Mexican hooker. Of course he may adore Mexican hookers, but check first...

Most men don't like women to wear too much make-up. In particular, skin should be left as natural as possible. Foundation is something on which to build a house, not a romantic relationship. Eyes are also important. Mascara may not be your idea of sex in a bottle, but a suggestive, wide-eyed glance can be one of the biggest aphrodisiacs of all.

When it comes to men, women don't like to see them in make-up at all. We all want intimacy, but it's not your skin-care tips we want to share – something more along the lines of beauty sleep, perhaps?

cosmetics

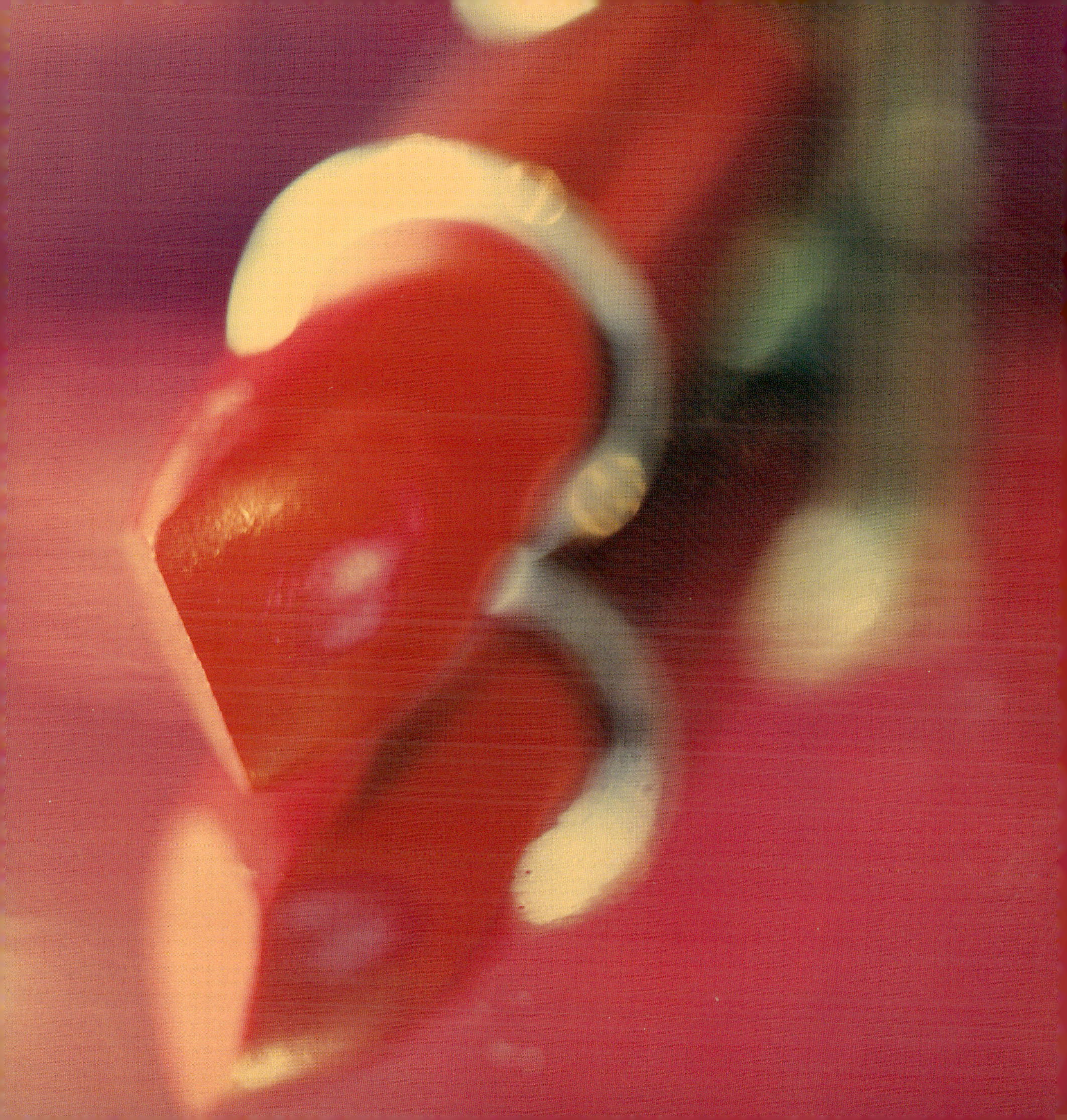

As the founder of ***Cosmopolitan*** magazine, Helen Gurley Brown, said, 'When the going gets tough – buy shoes.' No matter if your womanly hips are threatening to invade a neighbouring country, your shoe size remains girlishly the same and the assistant doesn't faint whenever you mention it.

But whereas a woman buys shoes when she needs cheering up or wants to transform herself magically into a sex symbol, a man buys shoes when his old ones wear out.

This is a shame, because no matter how pleased he might be to see us, the first thing many women look at in a man is further south that you might imagine.

While a great pair of shoes will not ensure you a place in anyone's bed, bad shoes will almost certainly banish you to the spare room of love. For men, anything white, grey or patent is out. Remember, guys – Elvis *is* dead. The rule is to keep footwear simple and unfussy.

Women have it easy. Every one of us surely has at least one pair of extravagant shoes hidden at the back of our wardrobe – bought at a time when we thought our toes were fat and we were definitely going to lose weight – but don't they look divine? This is the time to unearth them.

You don't have to stand up in them. Their function is purely ornamental – just cross your legs, arch your foot and purr. Most men are suckers for a stiletto heel. Not without reason did Germaine Greer call them 'f*** me heels'.

A friend who recently bought a pair of green snakeskin Gucci boots with heels high enough to give her altitude sickness took them tenderly out of their tissue-lined box for my admiration and stroked them lovingly. 'Tart's shoes,' she said with a happy sigh.

Exactly.

shoes

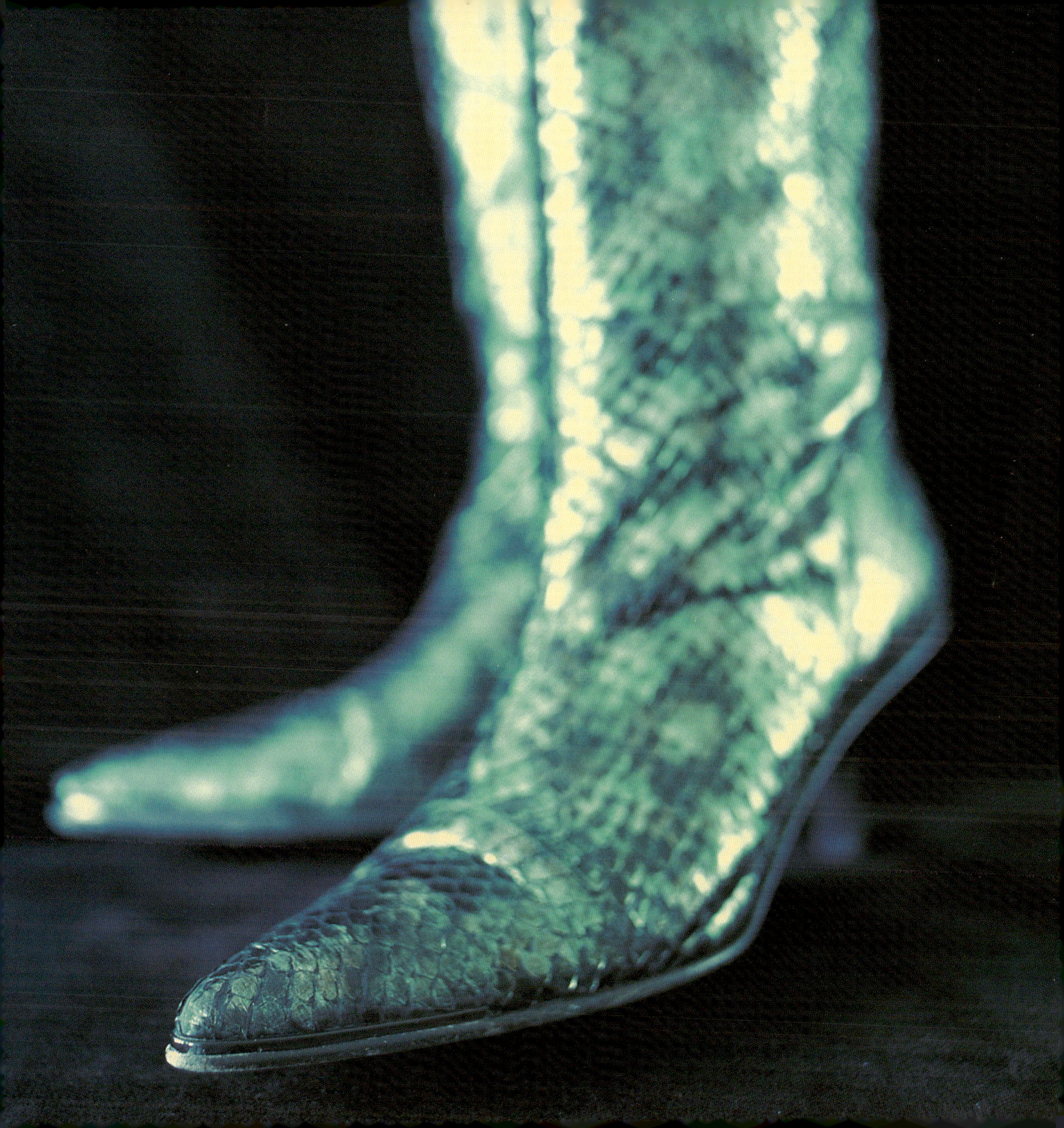

decoration

It's not just what you wear on your body that can make you look inviting, but also what you put next to your skin. Many men find the contrast between bare skin and painted finger-nails very alluring. There are also some more adventurous forms of adornment than traditional jewellery. You either love it or hate it, but some people find discreet body piercing a big turn-on.

If a pierced navel doesn't appeal to you, tattoos are another controversial form of erotic decoration. Not many of us find it a useful social skill in a man that he can make the tiger tattooed across his chest roar with a flex of his pecs, but something small and tasteful on a firm, toned and rarely seen muscle can look attractive.

Anything containing the word 'mum' or the name of your last lover is, of course, so out that you might as well sign yourself up for that second term in the Foreign Legion now – at least the desert robes will conceal the horror underneath. Similarly, curvaceous bikini-clad women should be *in* your arms, not tattooed on them with dye.

However, the problem with a tattoo is that, unlike the man you brought back from your summer holidays, it's permanent. You can't change your mind if you don't like it or when the bluebird in full flight across your abdomen starts to flag under the strain of the few pounds you gained at Christmas. Laser treatment to remove an unwanted tattoo is expensive and not always successful.

Most girls, understandably, don't want to end up with arms like a sailor. What joy that there are now any number of fantastic ways to cheat. Fake transfer tattoos wash off in a few days and henna fades gently over a period of weeks. Henna looks spectacular, but whether or not it has spectacularly sexy results depends on what your designs are, and who you show them to.

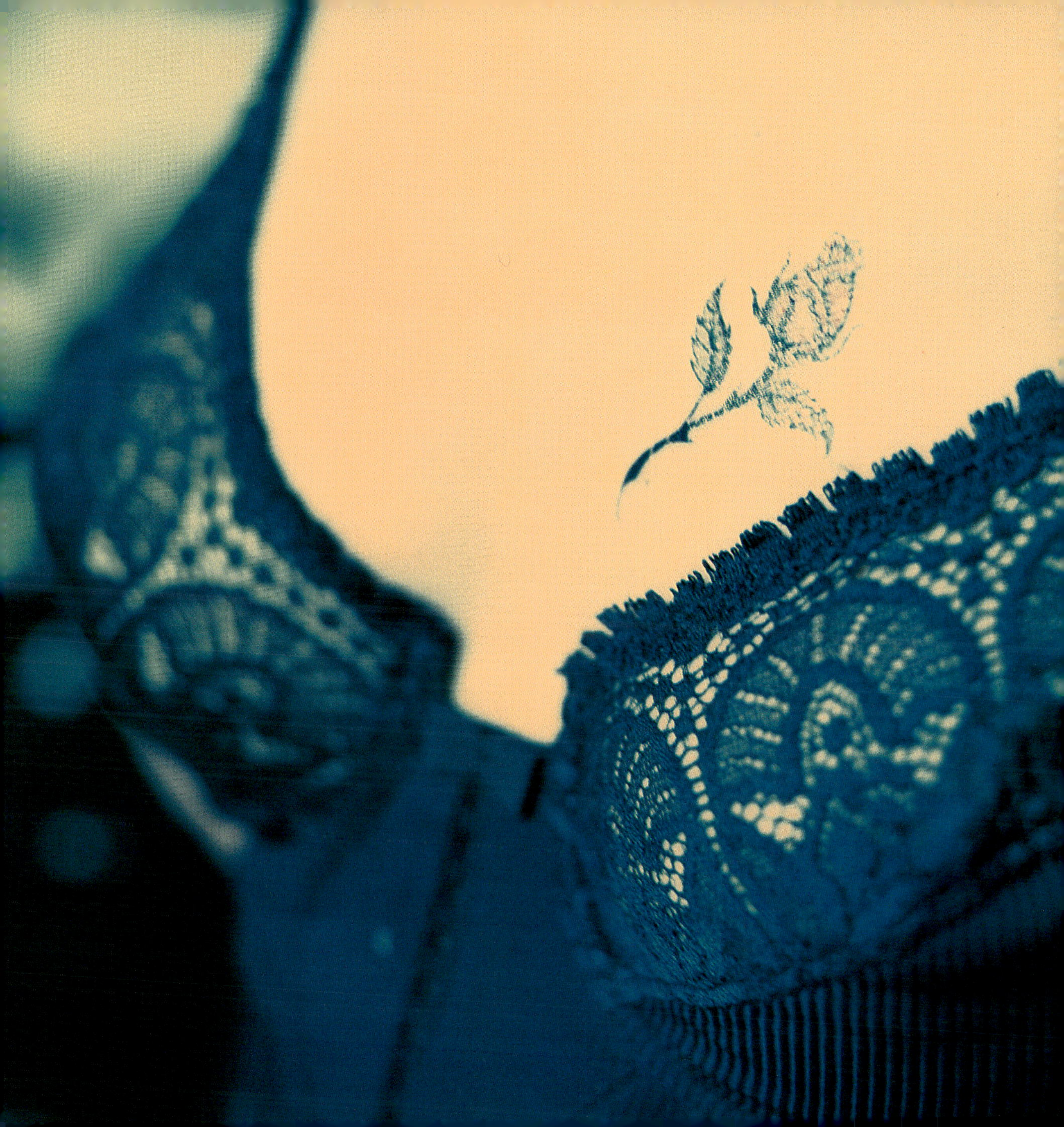

A man who knows his way around the kitchen is thought by many women to be supremely sexy. Isabel Allende in her book *Aphrodite* tells of being seduced by her husband's expertise with a frying pan, but although I appreciate a man who is good with his hands, juggling skillets does very little for me. A man who can cook is certainly impressive, but not if he exhausts himself over a hot stove in the process.

The current cult of cooking to impress has turned entertaining into more of a trial by dinner than a labour of love. Life is too short to peel a grape and if it's still true that the way to a man's heart is through his stomach, then we can all relax – it's not his stomach we're interested in. Some men find a woman in an apron too redolent of their mothers to be sexy and others, thank goodness, are happy to eat out.

Several of my women friends think that being taken out to dinner is tantamount to foreplay. Being expected to clear up the kitchen after their lover has cooked an elaborate meal is less of a turn-on.

There is a difference, however, between casual cuisine and indifference. Even if you buy the salad ready washed and the food microwave fresh, dress it up a little. Set the table with flowers, light candles and use elegant wine glasses.

Eating together is such an intimate act that some women find it easier to take all their clothes off and sing the first three bars of 'Hey Big Spender' than to swallow a morsel of food in front of someone they are still getting to know. Ply such a woman with endless portions of lascivious, difficult-to-eat dishes and be ready to accompany her when she bursts into song.

dining

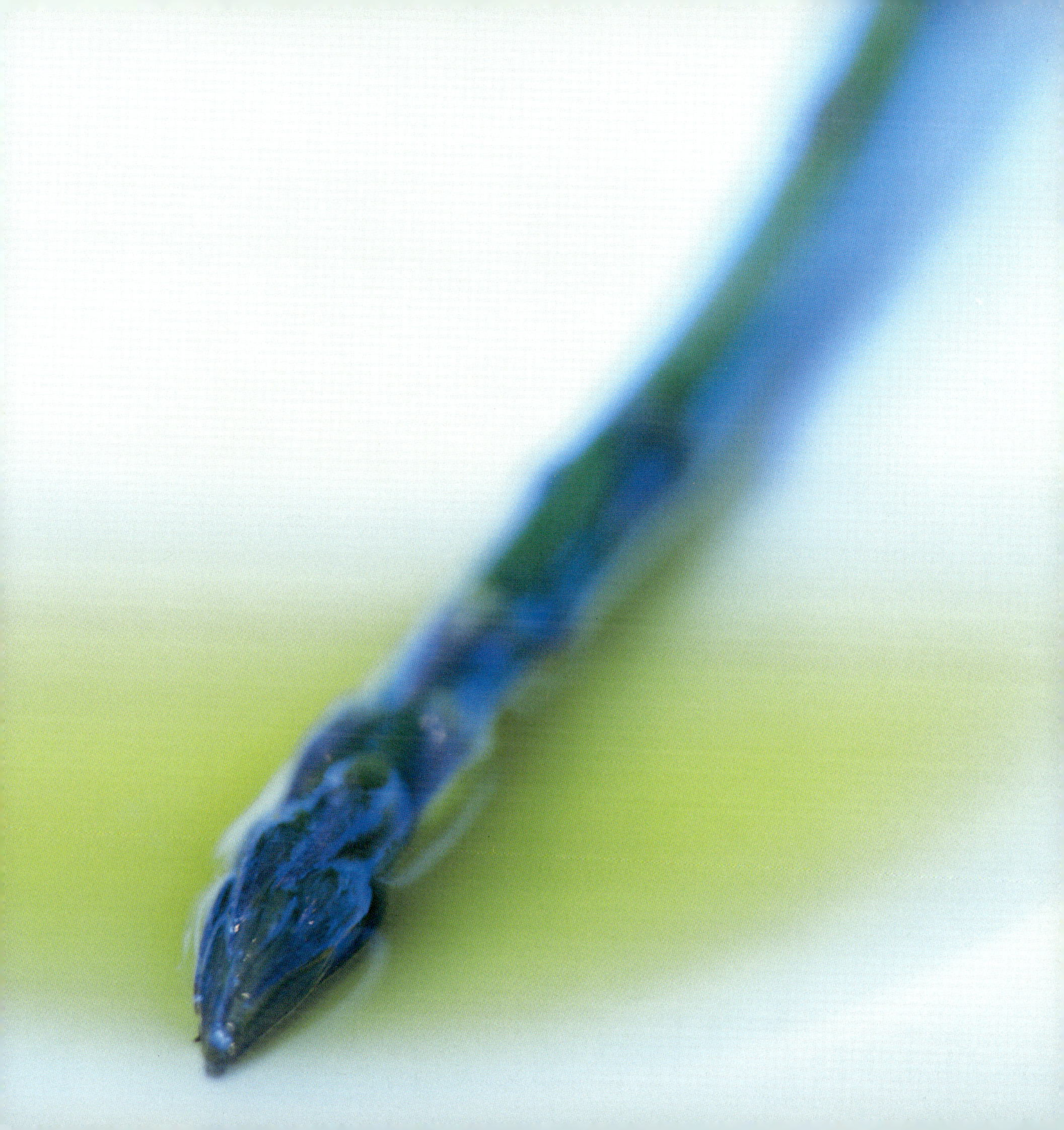

To get your partner into the right frame of mind for love you can begin by creating a seductive atmosphere. The old clichés are true – flowers, firelight, candlelight, soft music and a bottle of chilled wine go a long way towards encouraging passion. At the very least, clean sheets and a rapid tidy-up of the bedroom will indicate your amorous intentions.

In the Spike Lee film *She's Got to Have It* the heroine seduced her lovers in a room bare of everything except a bed and several hundred candles. As well as looking fantastic, candlelight is also very flattering. With no harsh overhead lighting to reveal those secrets you wish to share only with the bathroom mirror, you can relax and let yourself go.

If you use aromatherapy or scented candles, you can fill the room with pleasant fragrances at the same time as you light up your love life. You can also burn incense, or add a few drops of oil to the fire itself.

The room should be kept warm, but not tropical. You want to encourage your partner to shed garments, not five per cent of his body weight. If you insist on being seen as an intellectual you can leave copies of current non-fiction scattered across the coffee table, but it might be best to hide *Macramé Weekly* and *The Pigeon Fancier* under the sofa cushions.

Even for love in the afternoon, a bit of discretion with the lighting is advisable. First of all you don't want to shock the neighbours, and secondly strong sunlight will reveal just how much padding there is in your bra and where you bought it. Muslin, especially the coloured variety, can filter out the worst home truths and diffuse the light enough for you to leave your inhibitions on the carpet with the rest of your clothing.

setting the scene

It's not what you wear – it's how you wear it. A nice idea but, when it comes to seduction, just not true. Men in particular have endless dressing-up fantasies, but often it's your willingness to indulge them, rather than the idea itself, that they find most erotic. Some men go weak at the knees at the sight of a low-cut dress or even the vaguest glimpse of a bra through a sheer blouse, and stockings, unfortunately, continue to ring more bells than a campanologist's convention.

Stockings are hell. They are uncomfortable, archaic and not flattering to the fuller thigh, but what can I tell you – they work... The hold-up type act almost as well on the male libido as those with suspenders, but can make you look like a cross-dressing Michelin Man if too tight. Worse, if worn after a liberal application of body lotion, they will slide to a puddle at your feet when you least expect it – for example, in the middle of the street when leaving the Chelsea Hotel at four in the afternoon. Stockings are like fine wines – they don't travel and should be kept in a dark place until brought out for special occasions.

The art of dressing up lies in finding a way to hint at the glories to come while still leaving something to the imagination. Some women think that leather trousers are the male equivalent of the Wonderbra, while others say that a man in a dinner jacket is sex on legs. And while on the subject of legs – get thee behind me, tartan. Only Prince Charles wears a kilt as if it were some sort of upper-class leisure wear. Knees and plaid don't mix. A good pair of jeans will say more about you, and the contours of your derrière, than anything else. And if any woman says that she is just looking at your bottom to check out the label – she is *so* not telling the truth.

dressing up

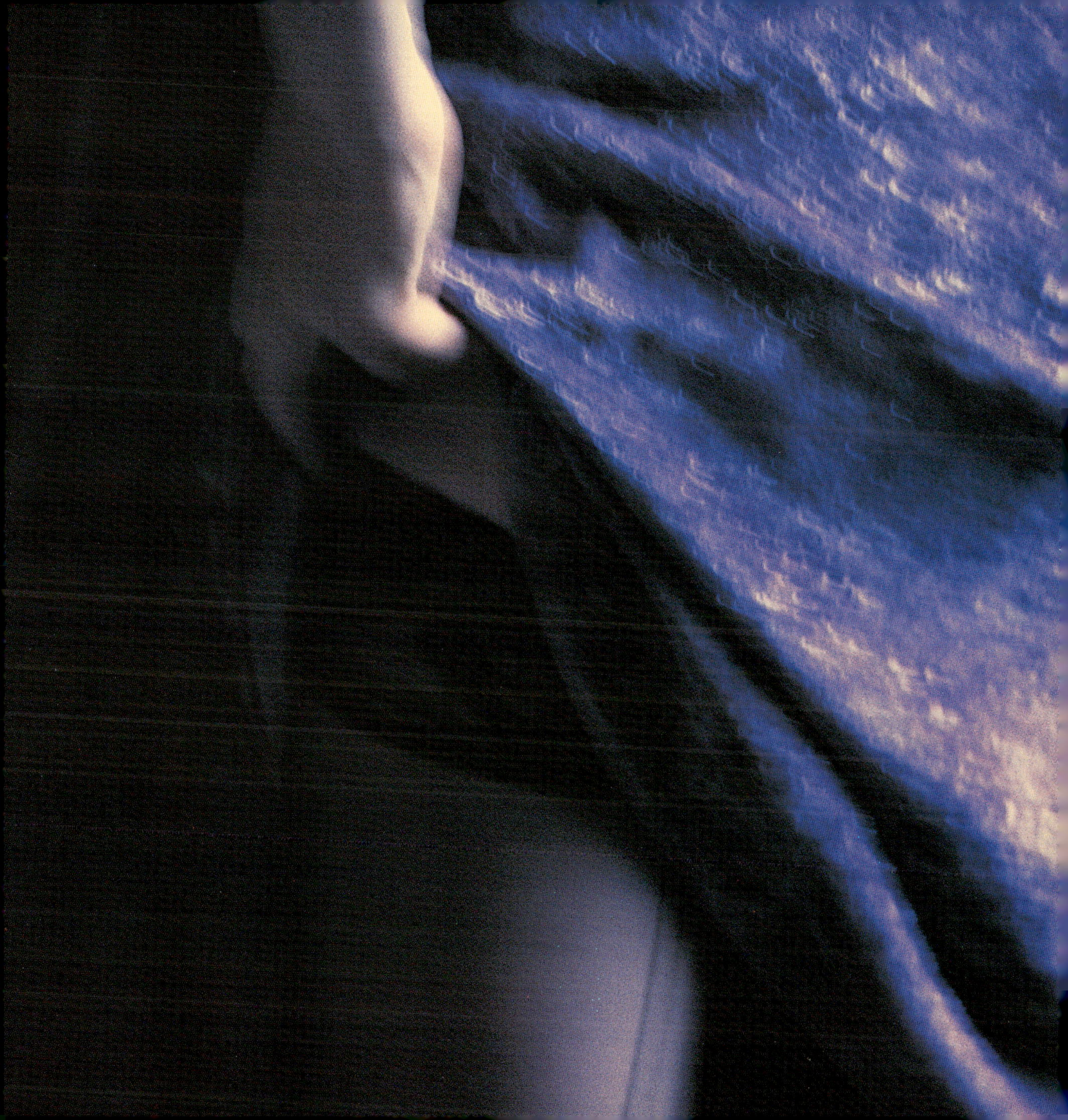

Men like women with long hair. It's not one of the ten commandments of sexual attraction, like thou shalt shave thy legs – it's just a preference. Quite a strong preference. But a woman having any hair at all is enough for some men, and God bless them.

Undoubtedly, long, healthy, flowing locks are irresistibly attractive but, just like a Gold American Express card, we can't all have them on demand. Long greying hair can be ageing on a woman and hint that she is trying vainly to hold on to her youth at a time when she should be reaching either for the scissors or for the rejuvenating power of hair colour. Of course, on some women, it's incredibly sexy, but it's important to know which category you fall into. The condition of the hair is also significant – better short than frayed at the ends.

This is a lesson men have learned better than women. The current trend towards shaven heads as a disguise for incipient baldness can be immensely sexy. Every time I meet a man with closely cropped hair I see Bruce Willis, barefoot, minus his shirt, running through a burning building – and since I like Bruce Willis (within those strict parameters), I'm fascinated.

However, I also like Daniel Day-Lewis with his long hair bouncing down his back, stripped to the waist and running through the North American countryside in a loincloth. I find myself asking if the problem of a bad hair day could be solved, not by a visit to the hairdresser, but just by taking off your shirt?

I'd guess it works for women too.

hair

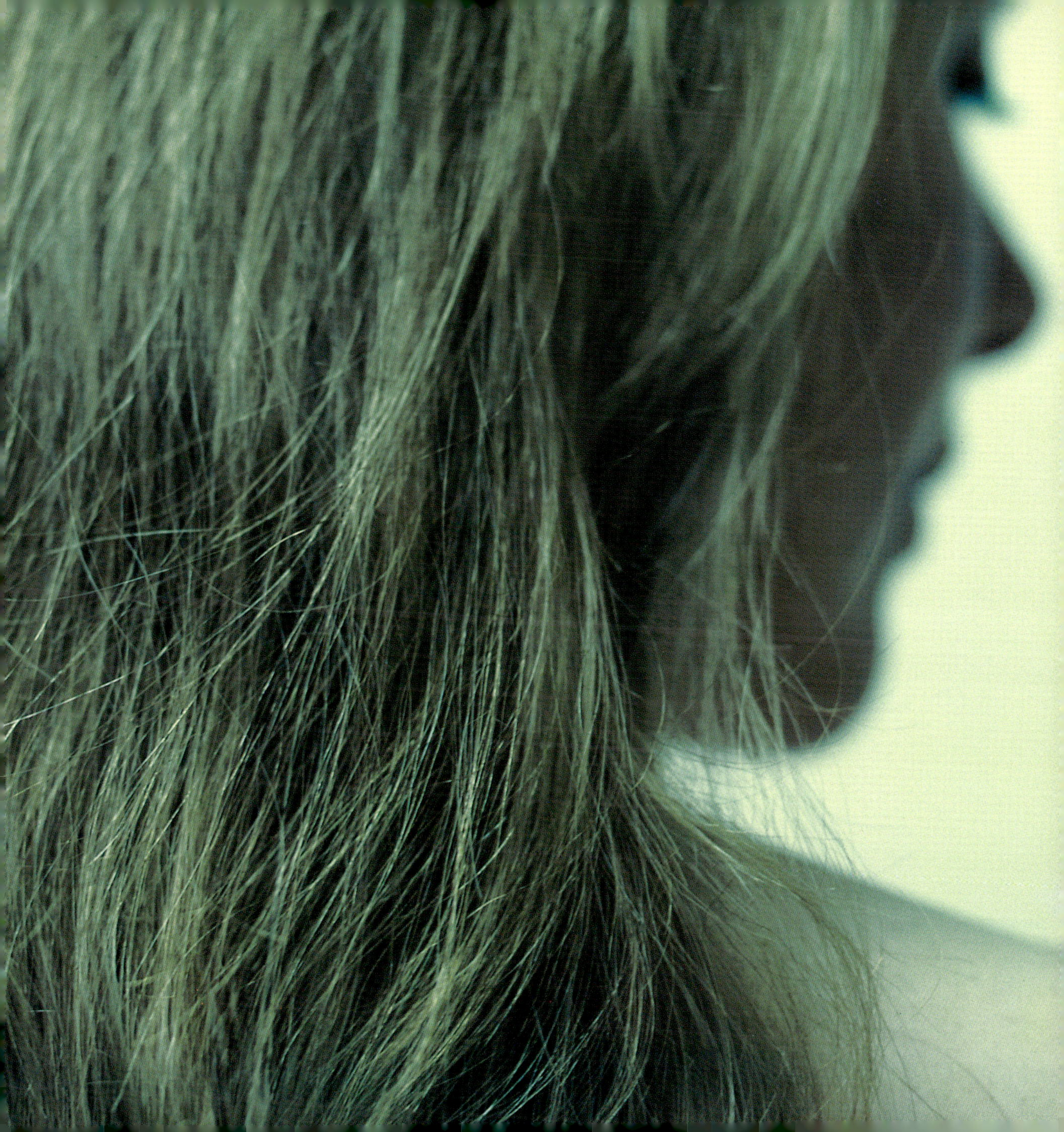

Although fur undoubtedly looks best on its original owner, there is nothing like the voluptuous feel of its decadent warmth against your skin. Thankfully, with the introduction of some wonderfully luxurious fakes, nowadays we can cheat. The only one who need go naked in order to enjoy the warmth and sensuality of fur is you.

Some men long to meet a woman wearing a fur coat, a pair of stockings and nothing in between. It's my suspicion that those fur-lined raincoats actually have very little to do with keeping you dry when it's raining outside. However, even those of us with Tarzan and Jane fantasies might find a man in a tiger-skin jockstrap just one fur too far. There are some things best left for the office party, and this is one of them.

One of my friends finds the delicate touch of a single feather deeply erotic, but beware of ticklish partners. You may want to rouse the slumbering beast in your lover, not play decoy ducks underneath the eiderdown. Instead, buy some slinky satin sheets, throw a fake bear skin across the bed and plump up your pillows. Or drape yourself languidly on a fake fur rug in front of an open fire and watch out for sparks.

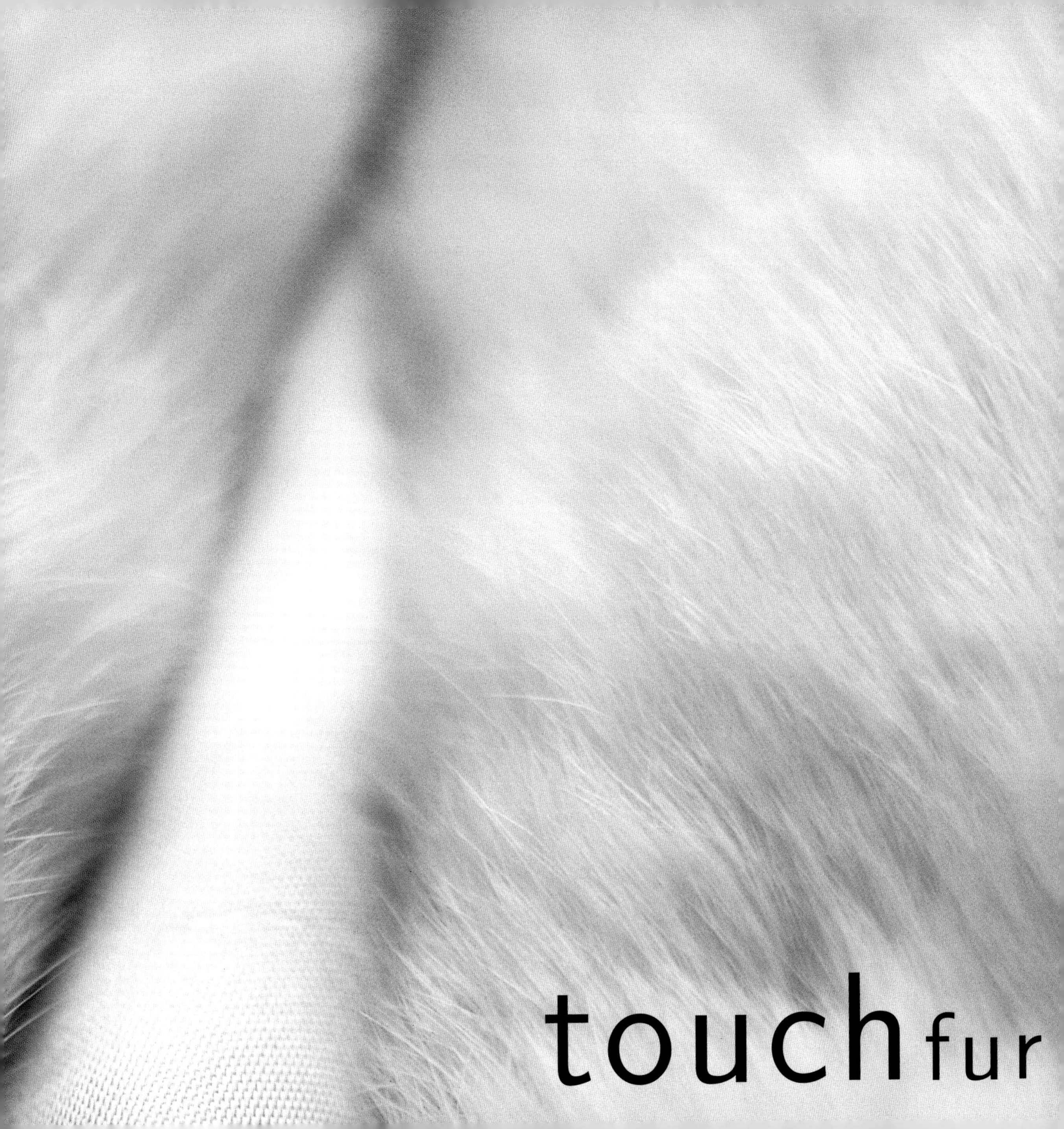
touch fur

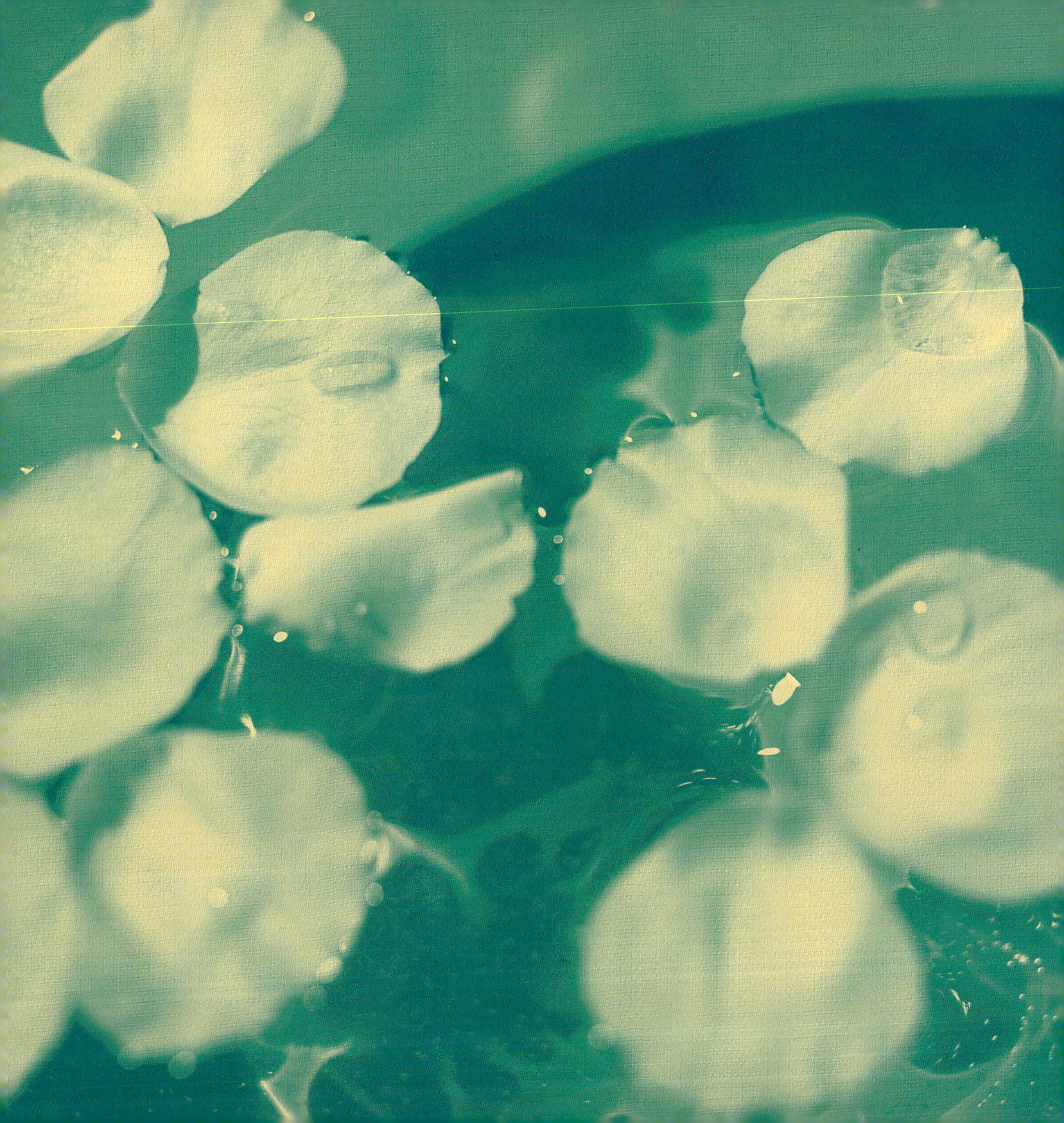

Maybe it's the feeling of returning to the womb, or perhaps just the sheer sense of luxury, but floating in sweetly scented water is the closest thing to heaven on earth. Cleopatra is said to have bathed in milk, which sounds worryingly pungent given the warmth of the Egyptian climate. However, modern life can be equally quixotic. When Tom Cruise and his wife Nicole Kidman were staying in a London hotel, they apparently filled the tub with champagne. Unfortunately the chambermaid thought the water had gone cold, and emptied it.

If you can't run to Tom Cruise, or even champagne, don't despair – there are any number of wonderful bath products on the market. Do make sure that the scent fits the occasion – this is not the time to soak that old sports injury in eucalyptus and arnica. And although the man in your life will probably be delighted to join you in a bubble bath, he may not relish coming out of the water smelling like free-sample day at the perfume counter. Alexander the Great was said to smell of violets, but not all men have the stature to carry this off.

Scented oils such as jasmine, rose maroc and sandalwood are a fragrant and sensual alternative. Use them sparingly – if it seems appropriate to sweep your partner out of the foam and into the bedroom, remember that bath oil is slippery. Make waves by all means, but tread carefully.

Anyone with even a rudimentary sense of romance can make bathing an erotic experience. Switch off the lights and burn a few candles. Chill the wine, pour some exotic bath essence into the water and dissolve. They used to urge us to save water by bathing with a friend, but in my experience, you don't have to be particularly friendly – just interested.

bathing

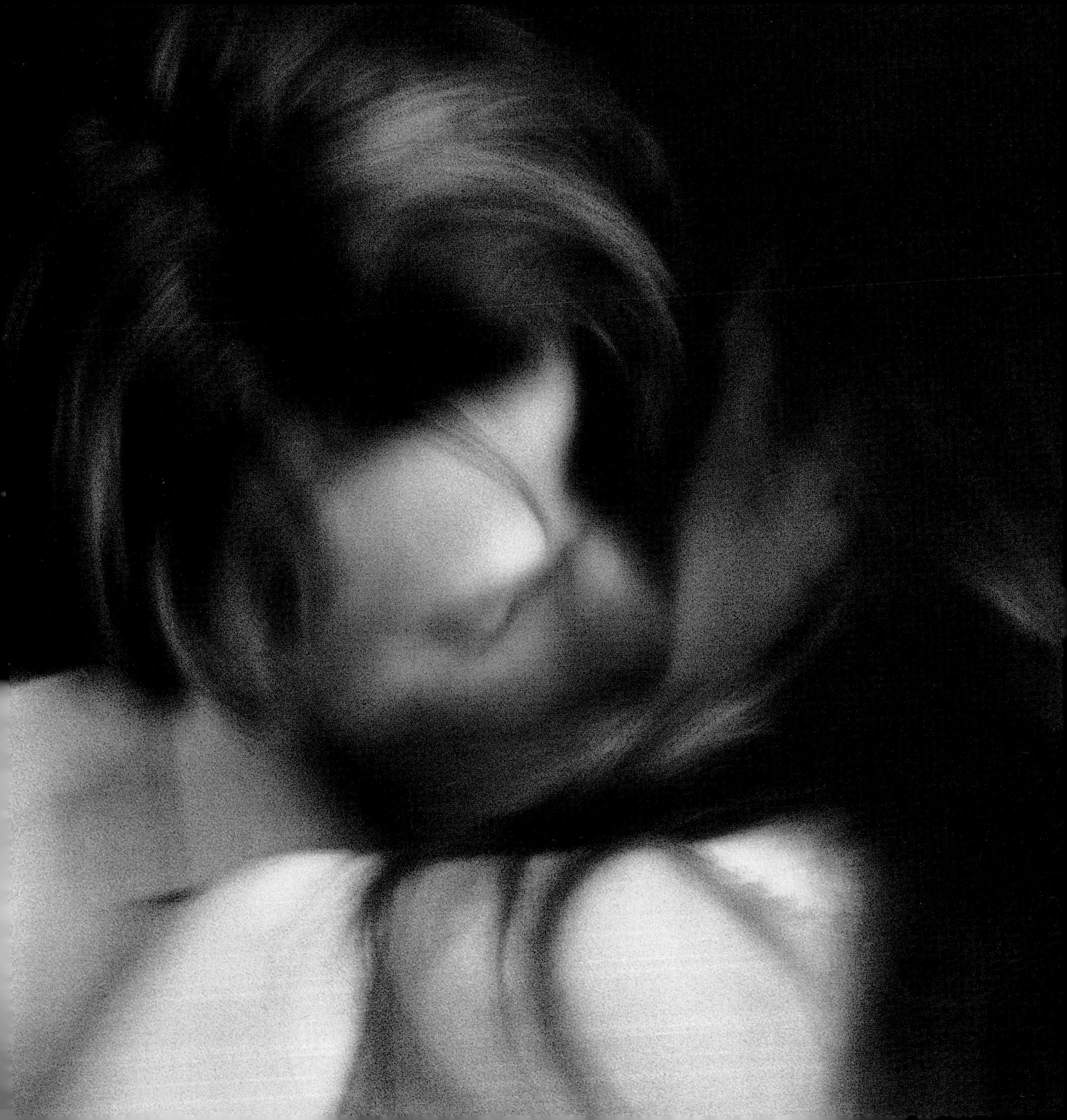

kiss

My friend Nancy recently complained that life as a single Californian girl was not the coital feast I imagined it to be. But it wasn't so much the sex she missed – it was the kissing.

Kissing is the single most deliciously erotic act. The feeling that there's an invisible cord pulling you both together, the warmth of someone's breath against your cheek, the softness of their lips, the melting uncertainty of wondering when, if, how, they are going to lean across and kiss you.

Some people seem to regard kissing as a sort of informal contact sport, but to me this is like playing football without bothering to score any goals. A kiss is not just a kiss – it is the primary sexual act and should inflame you into uncontrollable torrents of clothes-ripping lust. Convivial snogging is all very well, but while it's undoubtedly nice just to play the game, it's a lot more fun to get through to the finals.

However, because kissing is, in effect, a trailer for the big picture, you can tell pretty damn quickly if you want to hang around for the main feature. Some people definitely need to improve their kissing technique. There ought to be a kissing equivalent of boot camp, where you can send all those who could do with basic training. Remember that eyes, not mouths, are for drowning in, and while garlic and tobacco breath can bring a man to his knees, generally it's not for the right reasons. Shaving also helps – moustaches and beards turn some women on, but men are less fond of them, especially with lipstick.

The thing to do is to make time for lots of practice, in as many situations as possible. Meanwhile, Nancy has moved upstate and reports that her kissing famine is finally over.

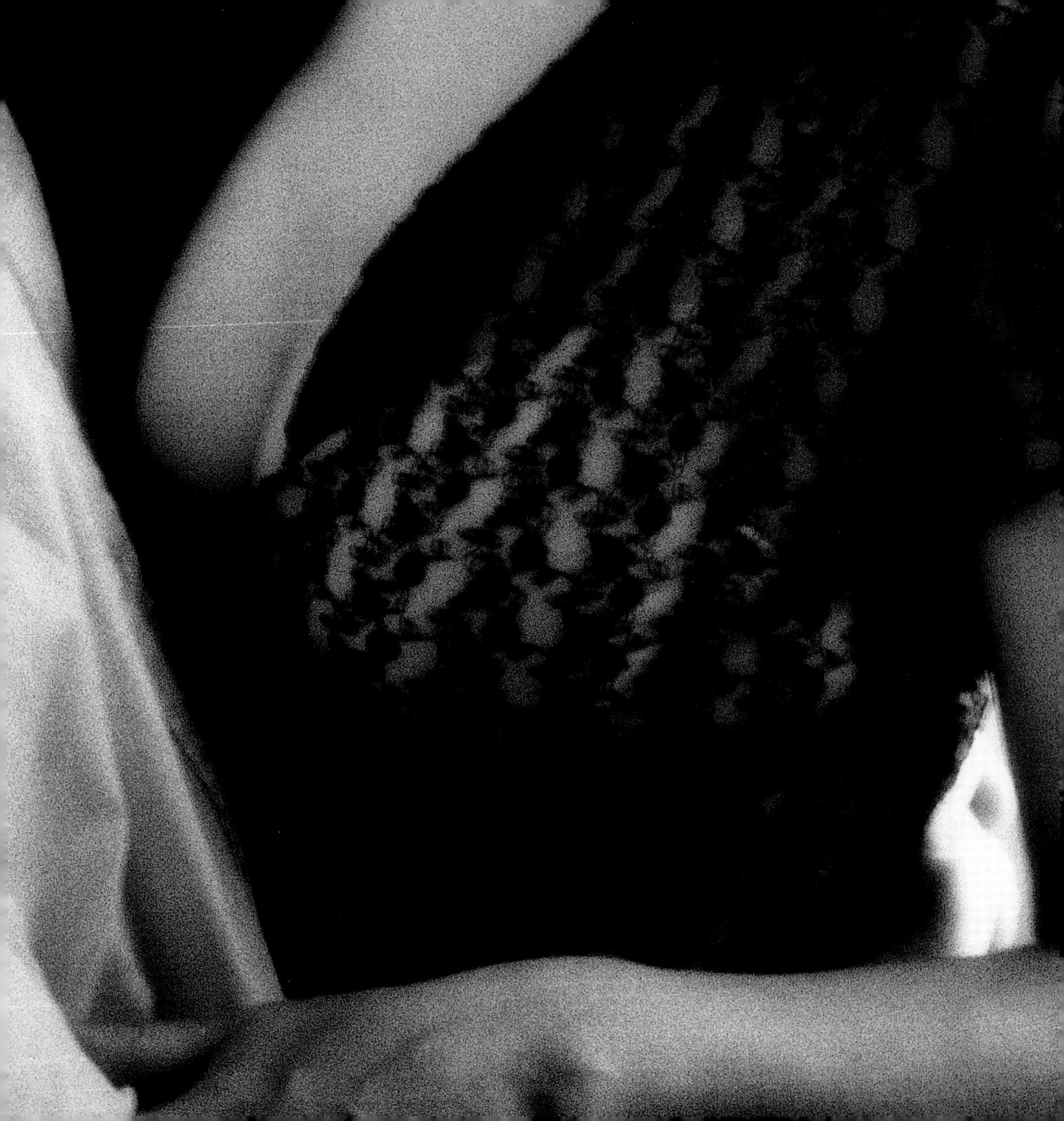

Dancing today seems to have evolved into a rather solitary pleasure: women dance with their handbags while men hug the edges of the dance floor as if they still believed that the world was flat and they were in imminent danger of falling off.

But some of us want domination, not domestication, and for that we need to go to the land of macho, stick a rose between our teeth and submit to a slow, pulsating beat. It's time to throw out our inhibitions and choose any one of those steamy dances from Latin America where you get to entwine yourself around a dusky stranger and practise safe sex with all your clothes on.

I went recently to a tango class fantasizing about finding a room full of tanned, lean Latin men, each with an impeccable sense of rhythm. Instead there was the instructor, a plump Argentinian with a paunch, a bandanna and Cuban heels – not a promising start to an evening of passion. He pressed my hand against his chest and ordered me to lean on him. Then the music surged and I was gone – swept away on a tide of tango. Suddenly, I was dancing with Al Pacino in *Scent of a Woman*.

Now it could be that I have an over-developed imagination that allows me to blank out reality, or perhaps there really is something incredibly sexy about being led around the floor by a confident man who knows just where he wants you, and when.

If this all seems too much for you, at least learn how to shuffle intimately around in a circle without stepping on your partner's toes. If she closes her eyes and is blessed with my powers of imagination she won't notice the difference. When she starts calling you Al, you're on the right track.

danc

For most of us the touch of smooth, clean skin is supremely erotic. Flushed skin hints at sexual arousal and tanned skin gives us an exotic, healthy look.

Woman are biologically designed to have less body hair than men, but we also exaggerate the sexual difference between us and our more hirsute partners by using oils and lotions to soften the skin, as well as various forms of medieval torture involving tweezers and hot wax.

Men, on the other hand, are permitted and in some cases even encouraged to flaunt their body hair. Many women like a man to look rugged, but if you are the possessor of a smooth, hair-free body there is no need to buy a chest wig or to tuck sprigs of parsley into the neck of your shirt. Not everyone wants to wake up next to the winner of a Yasser Arafat look-alike contest, especially when there's a full moon. At least a casual relationship with a razor will be appreciated by all kissable parts of your partner's skin.

However, it is sad but true that we are not all blessed with perfect complexions. Thankfully it isn't necessary to throw caution and all your clothes to the wind at the same time. The sexiest thing about skin is that you can reveal only small parts at a time. A carefully acquired tan from a bottle rather than the Côte d'Azur can disguise many of a woman's imaginary flaws, and she can always concentrate on her best points by opening a few buttons on her shirt or buying a revealing skirt.

Fake tans on men are bad news, as are shirts unbuttoned anywhere near the navel. A man over 50 is better off doing up a few buttons and getting a good night's sleep. Even for those women who like a bit of rough, growling will not help. Just gaze at her lovingly and tell her she's beautiful – she won't care if you look like King Kong.

She might even like it.

ski

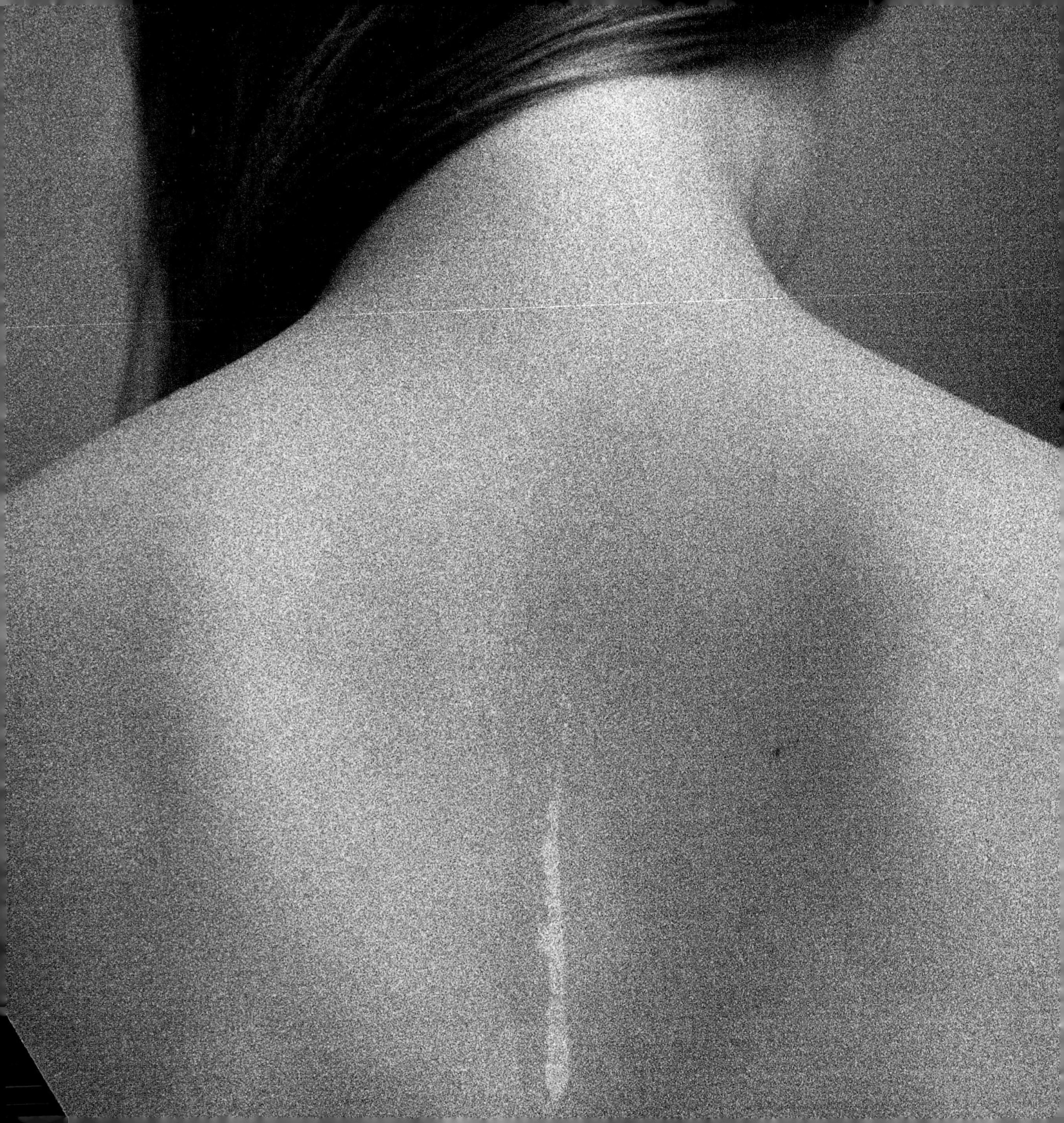

massage

I once knew a man, a judo black belt, who claimed to have 'magic' hands. His massages, he insisted, were out of this world, and he was right. They were firmly in the world of sports injuries, locker rooms and large women from Eastern European countries who do terrible things to your body with medicated liniment – the poor man had confused massage with physiotherapy and it was *not* erotic.

Bear this in mind when you decide to give your partner a massage. Forget those martial-arts films where high-kicking women make chopping motions across your back. Don't pummel the skin. Clapping and patting are fine for ponies and friendly dogs, but if you want to make your lover pant this is not the way to achieve it.

When massaging your partner, think about the journey, not what you are going to do when you get there. We all know where our major erogenous zones are, but you don't need to rush towards them with the same fervour as a child races into the sea. Take a walk along the beach first; enjoy the sun and frolic in the sand dunes before you even dip a toe into the surf.

A sensual massage uses stroking and kneading movements. Don't be too clinical about it – the aim is sensual, not medical. Use just enough scented massage oil or body lotion for the particular area you are concentrating on – and on the more tender parts of the anatomy, be sensible. Anything likely to sting or irritate is obviously not going to arouse your lover, except perhaps to send him or her in search of something with which to hit you over the head. Repeatedly.

Firm but gentle movements are those most likely to stimulate. Apart from the obvious areas, there are sensitive points along the inside of your arm right down to the tip of your middle finger. The front of the thigh to the tip of the knee is very responsive to touch, as is the area around the lower back and the nape of the neck. The feet are also loaded with nerve endings and give an intense feeling of relaxation when rubbed. There are numerous books which deal with the subject in detail, but hell – you really don't need absolute precision. Who is going to complain? They should be so drugged with the delicious feel of your hands that they are hardly going to tell you you've missed a bit.

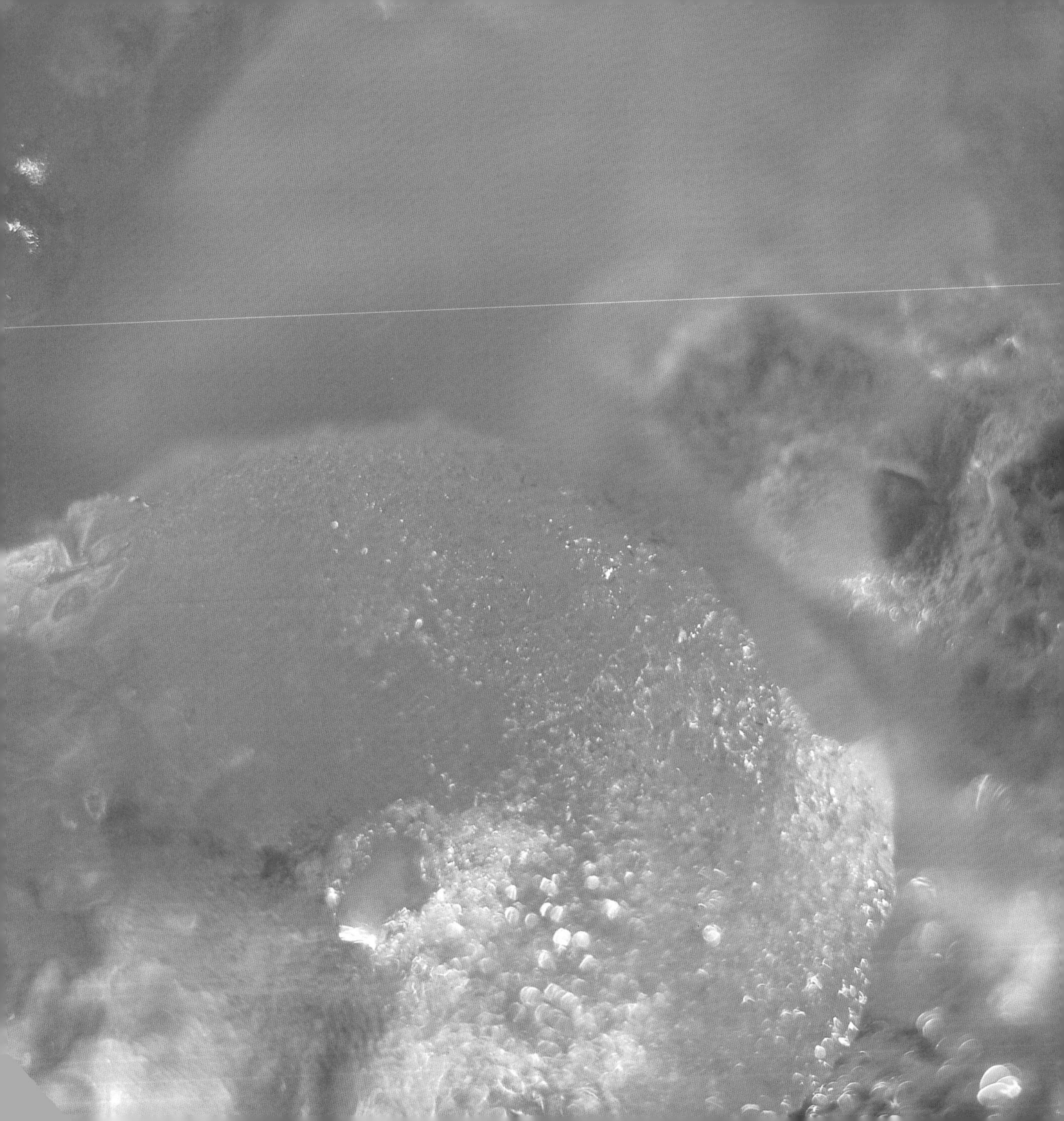

To be sensual, it has to be tactile, lush and luxurious. Silk and satin, fire and ice, the feel of the sun against your back, the stroke of a feather down your spine or the melting sensation of a snowflake on your tongue – any of these can be a sensual experience.

Silk and satin are at their most voluptuous when worn, and heavy satin sheets are a sensualist's dream. However, if the temperature is anywhere except in the high eighties, frankly, you are in for a rude shock. As well as being slippery, silk and satin make for cold bedfellows. They feel exquisite against your skin, but only once you've acclimatized to the sudden chill.

Plain white Egyptian cotton sheets, sent to the laundry for extra crispness, are more forgiving in the winter yet cool enough to withstand the most heated exchange in the summer. An added benefit is that you don't slide out of your lover's arms on to the floor at the other side of the bed. Velvet is another fabric which is rich, warm and so tactile that it begs to be touched.

However, sensuality is not defined merely by the objects surrounding you. Sometimes the very atmosphere can be erotic. Turkish baths and balmy steam rooms can initiate deeply languorous, seductive feelings, while the Scandinavians roll around in the snow after a warm sauna to invigorate themselves.

The thought of leaping from a hot, pine-scented cabin into a snow drift may not make you sizzle with desire, but it certainly puts the chilly satin sheets into some sort of perspective. For the less intrepid of us, ice cream needn't come with a bowl and a spoon. Alternatively, there are a lot of things you can do with an ice cube before you need worry about frostbite.

sensuality

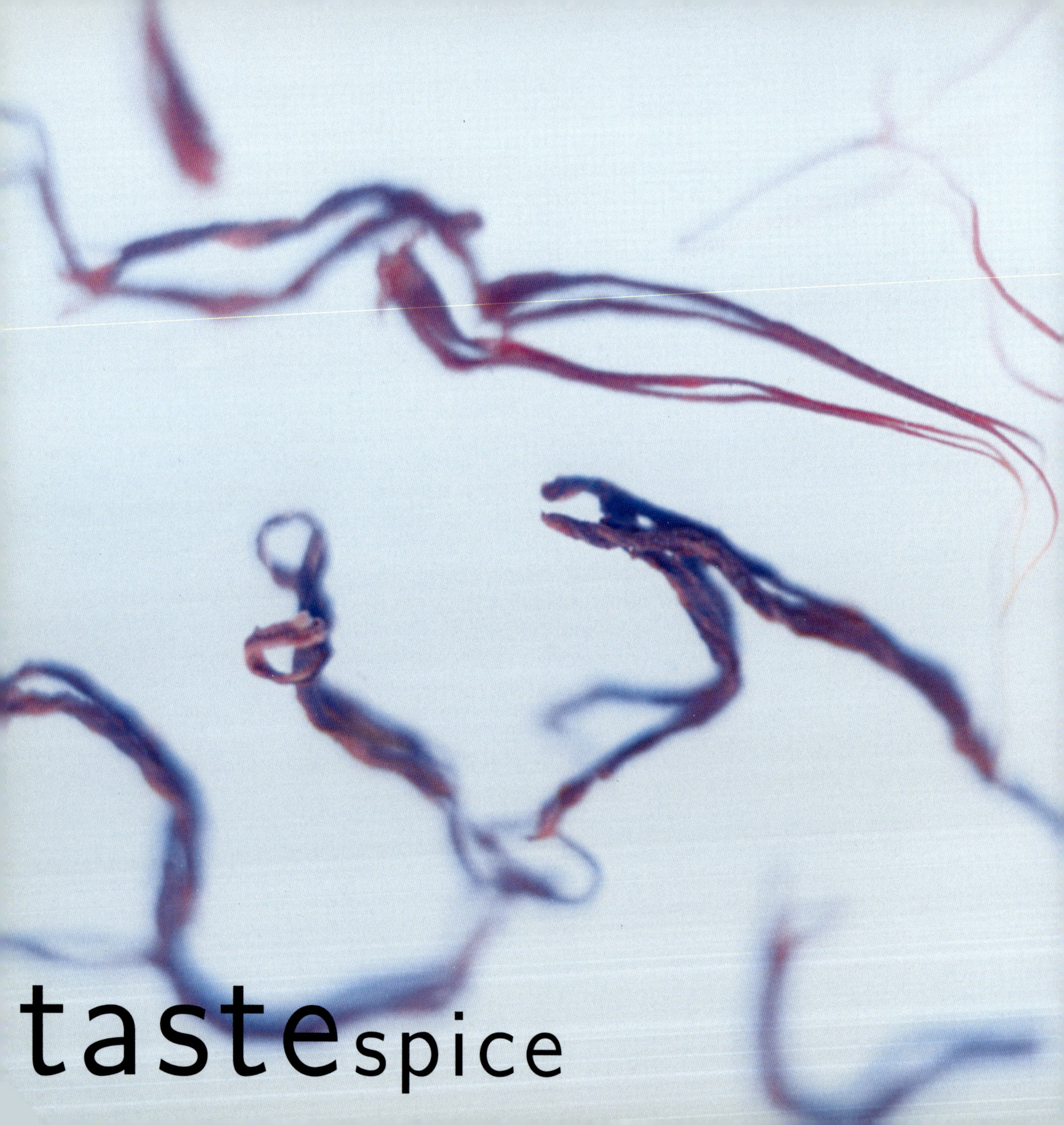

taste spice

There may well be some ulterior motive when your partner offers to take you out to dinner at an Indian restaurant, because spices have long played an important role in adding flavour to your love life as well as your food.

According to legend, King Solomon seduced the Ethiopian Queen Makeda by promising not to touch her unless she first took anything belonging to him. He then prepared a banquet of hot, spicy food and, when she tried to quench her thirst from his water jug, demanded payment in kind.

I think Solomon might have had to be a little more persuasive after a night at the local tandoori, but those eastern spices do contain their own promise.

Saffron – the pistils of the saffron crocus – has a very delicate flavour and is used more as a food colouring than as a seasoning. Despite this it is a traditional ingredient in numerous love potions, its staggering expense justified by its wondrous performance. Ginger, on the other hand, is a hot, pungent spice used throughout Asia and has the reputation of being a powerful and fiery aphrodisiac. Mulled wine – an infusion of ginger, cloves, nutmeg and cinnamon in some gently warmed red wine – is one way to warm your winter evenings and arouse your voluptuous nature. Nutmeg contains a mild hallucinogenic, cinnamon will warm the blood, while cloves have been used as an aphrodisiac in China since the third century. Even everyday condiments such as salt, pepper and garlic are said to inflame desire.

Many of these ingredients were traditionally used externally by mixing them to a paste and applying to pertinent areas. Now, I'm sorry, but I can't see it myself – garlic not only keeps away vampires but it can clear a room in five seconds. If you wear it as a moisturizer you may have perfect skin and a rod of steel, but believe me – you'll be fishing by yourself.

Far better to stick to using spices as a culinary seasoning. Ginger can be added to both beverages and foods. If you really insist you can mix it to a paste with honey and spread it all over your body to stir the fires of passion, but don't blame me if the blaze gets out of control.

fruits

Ever since Eve picked the forbidden fruit and led Adam into temptation, fruit has been associated with sin. Even today, when languishing in the hands of a lover instead of at the back of your refrigerator, any piece of fruit can take on the role of a seducer and send you rampant with desire.

Grapes and cherries are synonymous with sex. Small, round and bite-sized – who hasn't had the fantasy of reclining, scantily clad, on the chaise longue being tantalized by a bunch of succulent grapes – or is that just me? A word of warning, however: it may be erotic to lie back, lips apart, while your partner satisfies your hunger grape by grape, but not if you end up with a mouthful of seeds. You don't want to pad your cheeks with pips like a hibernating squirrel.

Strawberries, on the other hand, are the ultimate lovers' convenience food, combining all the attributes of size, colour and lusciousness, but without any worryingly large pips. They also come complete with little green detachable handles – useful for popping into eager mouths. The neurologist Alan Hirsch found that even smelling them could raise penile blood flow. So, for maximum benefit, forget the after-shave, guys, and just spray on a strawberry.

Taste apart, there is no getting away from the symbolic nature of food and its supposed aphrodisiac properties. However, forget about bananas – in this, if in nothing else, size really doesn't matter. Much like the muscular man who struts smugly around the gym in lycra shorts – bananas are case of overly blatant advertising.

Choose instead something exotic and deliciously juicy. Hindu literature suggests burying a mango under a tree trunk for six months and then making it into ointment. What a waste of time! Why not just eat it the way nature intended – with someone on hand to lick your fingers afterwards.

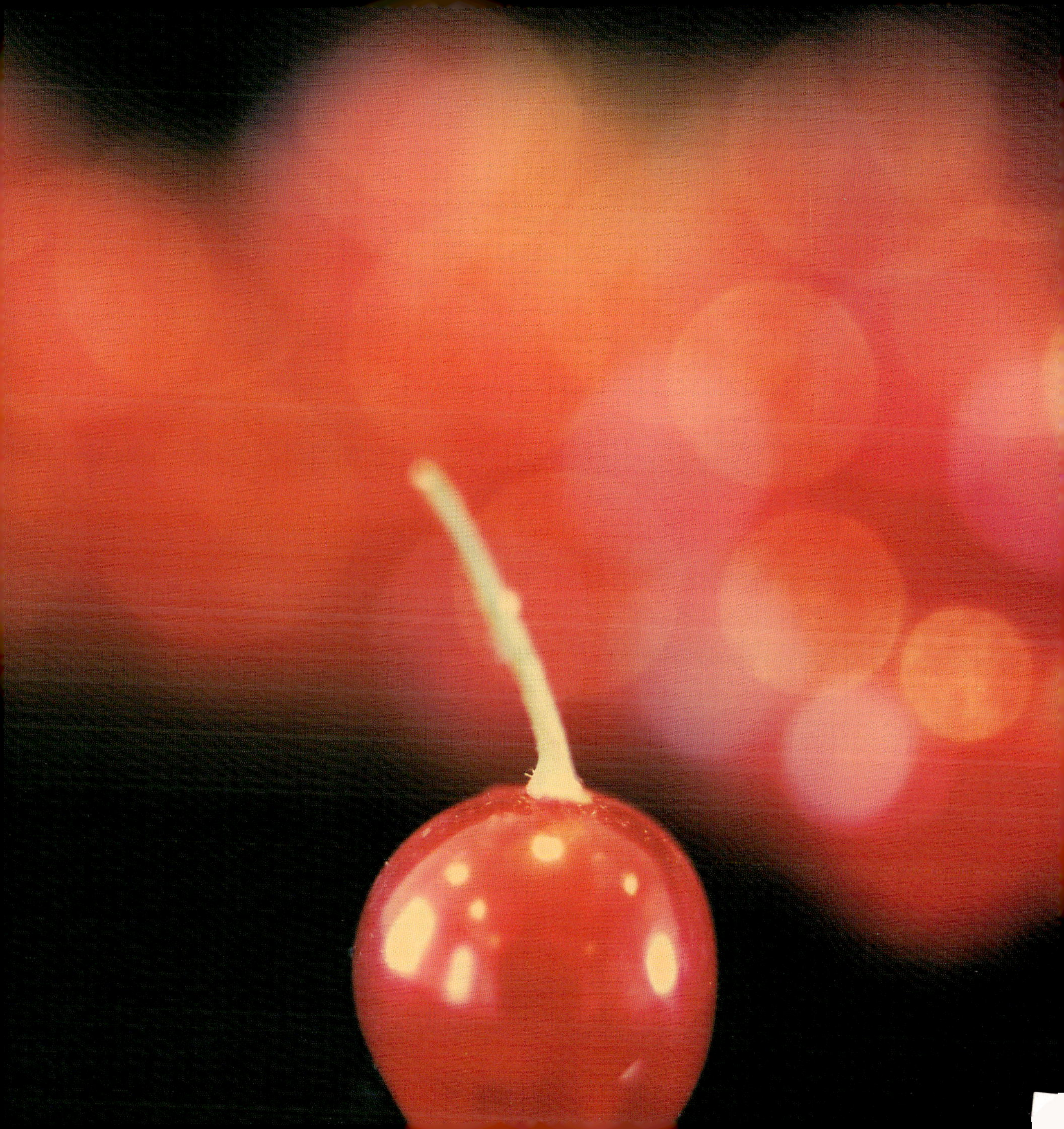

Figs are passion on a plate – plump, purple and ripe, they are the sexiest of all fruits.

Figs should always be fresh, not dried – you are targeting your libido, not your digestive system – and just pliant to the touch. No matter where it tells you to slice them open with a knife, never use anything sharper than a fingernail to peel back the skin.

What is this obsession with knives? Call me sceptical, but I defy anyone to feel erotic after watching a soft, succulent fruit being attacked by anything with a serrated edge. Perhaps this is why historically there are numerous taboos about knives and food consumption. At one time it was suggested that no round objects should be tackled with a knife and that even an orange should be peeled with a spoon, but this may be taking things a little far.

Forget stainless steel – use your fingers to delicately separate the folds and expose that wonderfully lush, pulpy interior. You can then tenderly nibble the flesh or, if the figs are really ripe, just wipe the skin and devour the whole thing, voluptuously.

Anyone who begins to slurp at this point has lost their credibility in the oral-gratification department. Served correctly, figs will surely invoke pure, unadulterated lust and provide you with boundless energy which, if you are doing everything properly, you are going to need.

Figs, apparently, also contain potassium – but, if you care a damn about that, then, darling, you have no soul.

fruits

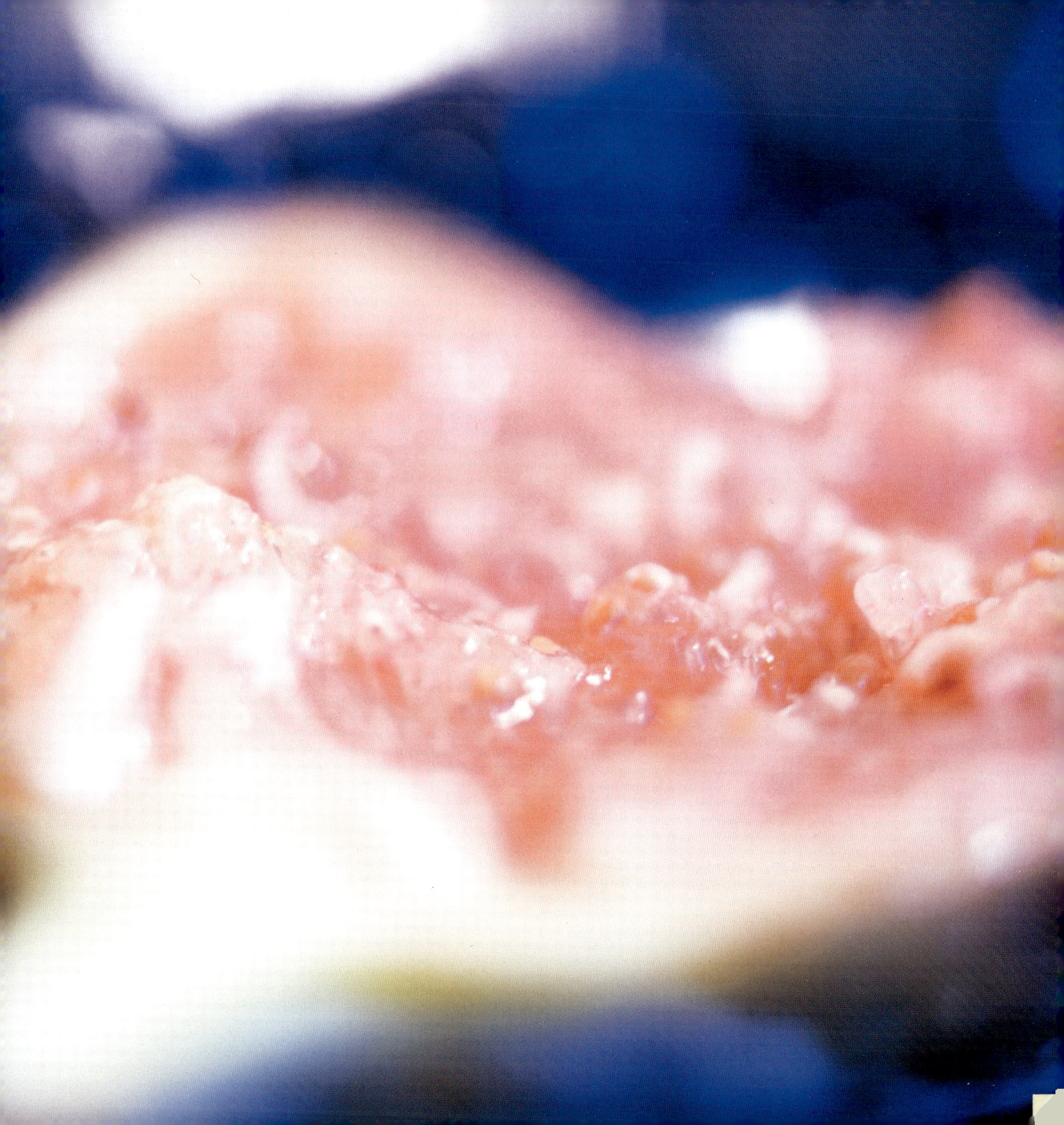

Throughout ancient cultures, plants, herbs and various disagreeable animal appendages have been used to increase sexual desire. Many traditional aphrodisiacs, such as rhino horn or ground antlers, are illegal, barbaric or just plain silly. Leave the poor animals' pointy bits alone and get your own. Other ingredients, such as the root of the mandrake plant or Spanish fly, a ground-up beetle, are highly toxic and likely to kill more than your libidinous urges.

The bark of the bois bande tree, which grows on Grenada, is infused in rum for several weeks to provide increased potency, while the yohimbine tree from Africa is used to stimulate a strong erection. Another effective aphrodisiac is a powder made of the white bark of the arjuna tree from India.

This is all very well if you have a tropical rainforest growing at the end of your garden and the foresight to allow enough time before seductions to make fortified boot-leg whisky. But if you start shaving bits off unidentified trees in your local park, you are more likely to go barking mad than boldly forth where no man has gone before.

Fortunately, there's always ginseng. This root, which grows in China and Korea, has been used medicinally for centuries. It is associated with virility and sexual performance, as well as general physical well-being. Unlike the more exotic ingredients listed above, you don't have to trek overland across distant continents to find it – a trip to the health-food store will suffice.

Guarana is another widely available substance and comes from the seeds of a South American shrub. It stimulates both the mind and the sexual appetite, while reducing hunger. This sounds like the ideal aphrodisiac, particularly if you need to do a spot of mental arithmetic while making love. In an overly precipitous lover, this skill may be more useful than you might think.

natural highs

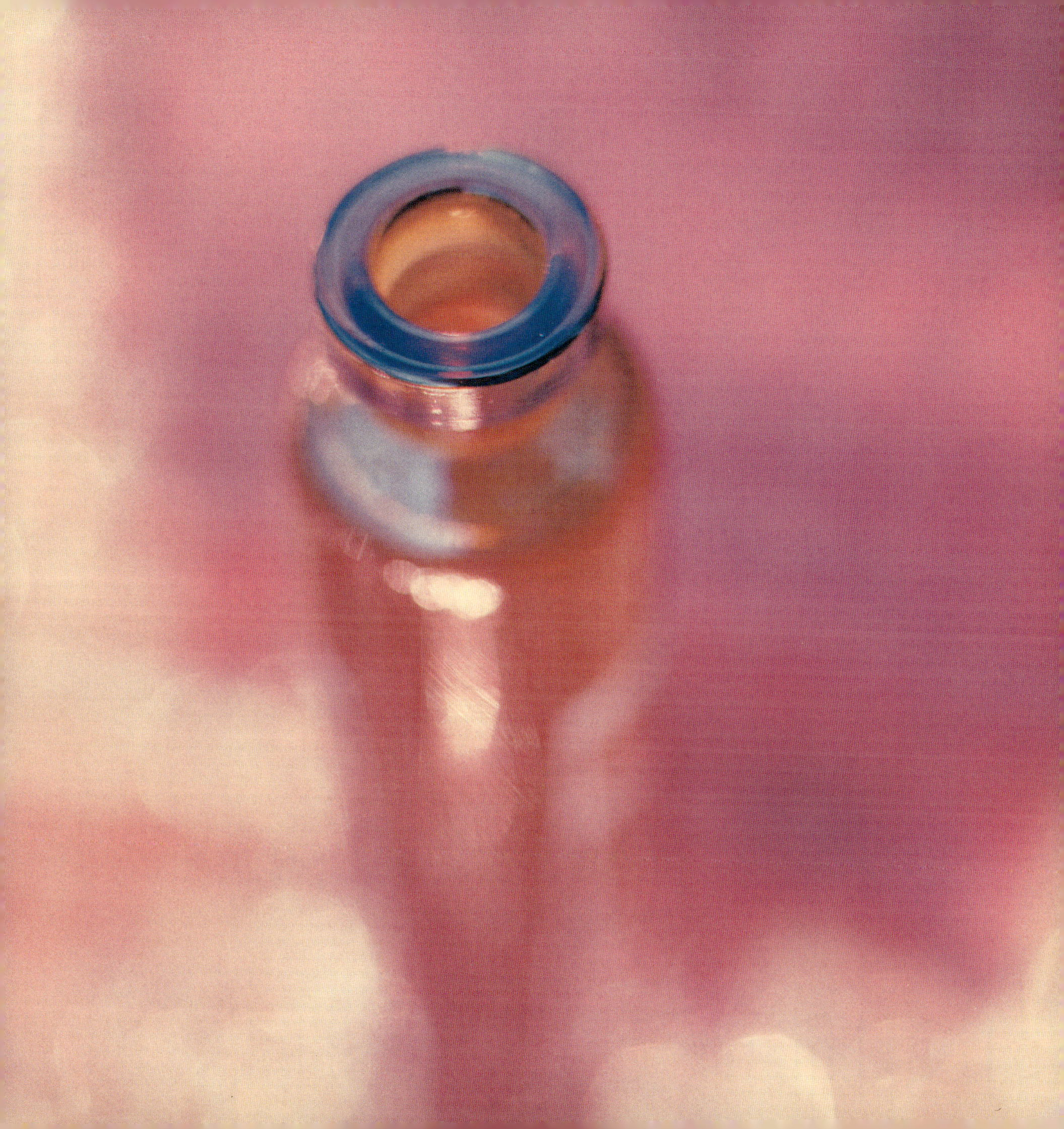

shellfish

Oysters are frankly and unmistakably erogenous. You would have to be blind to be unaware of the sexual symbolism of an oyster on the half shell. Anyone dense enough to miss it is probably more interested in train-spotting than sex. Buy him a pair of binoculars and eat the oysters yourself.

Shellfish of any sort – anything you have to use your fingers for, or that needs to be teased out of its hard, protective covering and devoured, is said to do for the libido what a Ferrari does for a middle-aged balding bank clerk. Suddenly your engine is throbbing and you're ready to go. Hopefully not from 0–120 mph in 0.3 seconds – we'll settle for a long stretch on the motorway at a steady 75.

Oysters have long been used to improve vigour and by eating them you are said to be advertising your readiness for prolonged bouts of love-making. However, my friend Amanda has another theory. She says that the reason oysters are so sexy is that they have the smell and tang of the sea. They also taste briny and have a sensual viscosity about them, so that any man who relishes the flavour and texture of a raw oyster has a built-in appreciation for the taste of a woman. Obviously, Amanda's husband is an oyster man, which probably accounts for her generally satiated demeanour.

Caviar, another expensive gift from the sea, is also supposed to promote desire. Beluga, Sevruga, Osietra – even the names slip off the tongue with the same ease as the caviar itself. The ultimate luxury food, caviar is said to have anti-ageing properties, too. It comes in small tins or, less expensively, pasteurized in vacuum-packed jars. Eat it with a small spoon, alternated with sips of champagne or vodka, and if you are not in heaven, you should at least be in the waiting room.

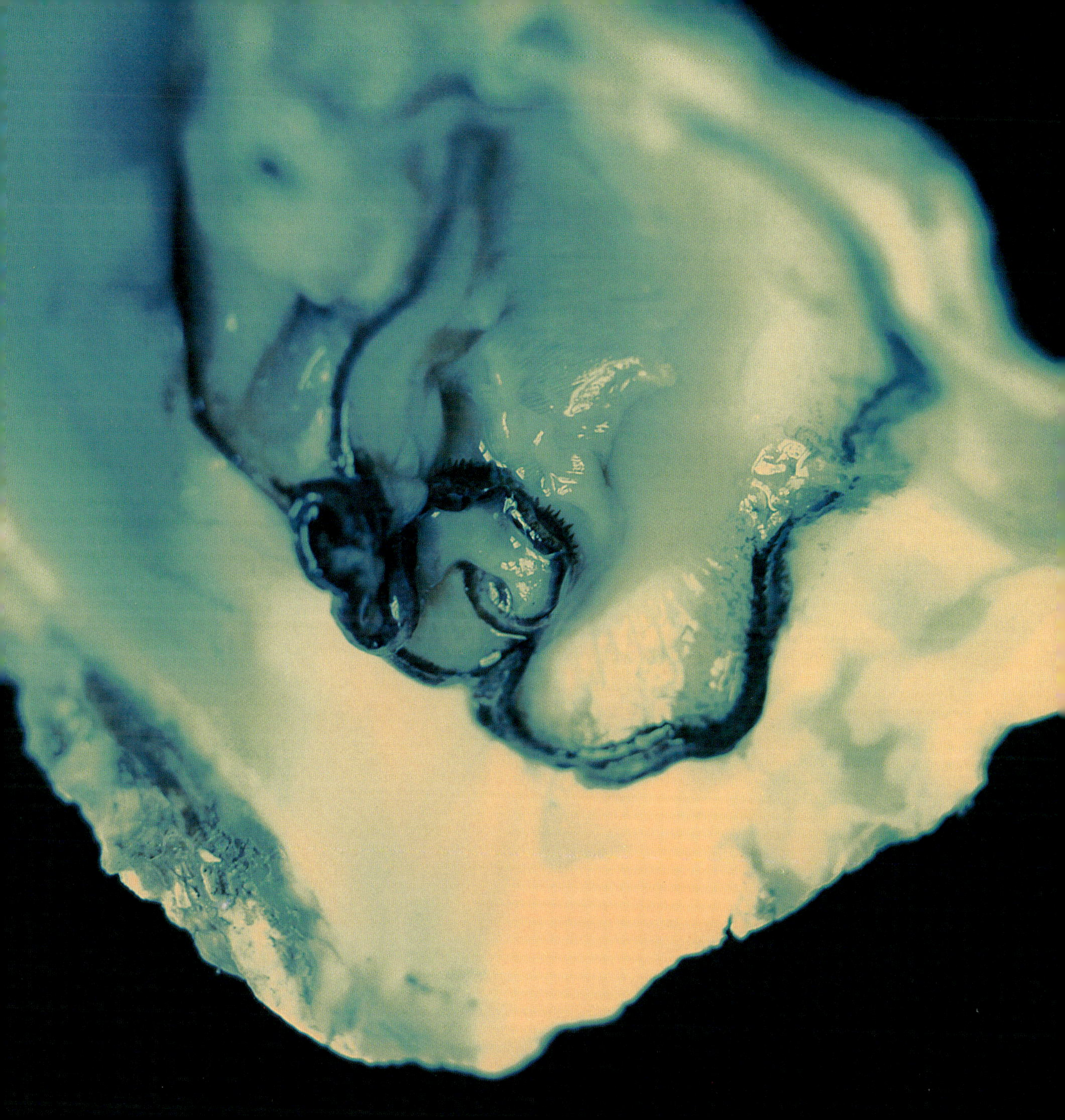

Chocolate, if not better than sex, is at least a good substitute. If you can have both then, as the Aztecs believed, chocolate must indeed be a gift from the gods.

Although originally served as an invigorating bitter drink, chocolate was introduced to Europe by the Spanish Conquistadors and sold in London coffee houses in its sweetened form as an alternative to gin. Its impressive reputation as an aphrodisiac probably derives from the direct effect chocolate has on the pleasure centres of the brain – it has been scientifically shown to raise levels of serotonin, which controls our moods, and to increase feelings of general well-being. For some women, a wedge of chocolate-frosted devil's food cake can replicate the sensation of blissful post-orgasmic satisfaction, thereby drawing even more parallels with sex – both pleasures are richly indulgent, but once satisfied, induce sleep.

Naturally, the way round this is to serve chocolate in modest quantities, especially for those sad people who see chocolate as fat instead of foreplay A tiny tart from a patisserie or one of those miniature boxes of sinful hand-made delicacies will whet your appetite but not completely satisfy it. When buying chocolate, small is beautiful, but you do need to part with some serious cash. No woman has even been successfully wooed by a box of inferior, day-glo soft centres – most of us appreciate a partner who knows his way around a box of Belgian truffles. The higher the content of cocoa solids, the better the quality of the chocolate. Real vanilla essence, a flavouring frequently added to cocoa, is itself an aphrodisiac and worth seeking out.

There are long-established rituals in sexual folklore involving certain parts of the anatomy and chocolate spread, whipped cream or even honey, one of the oldest aphrodisiacs of all. If you intend to invoke any of these – skip dessert.

chocolate

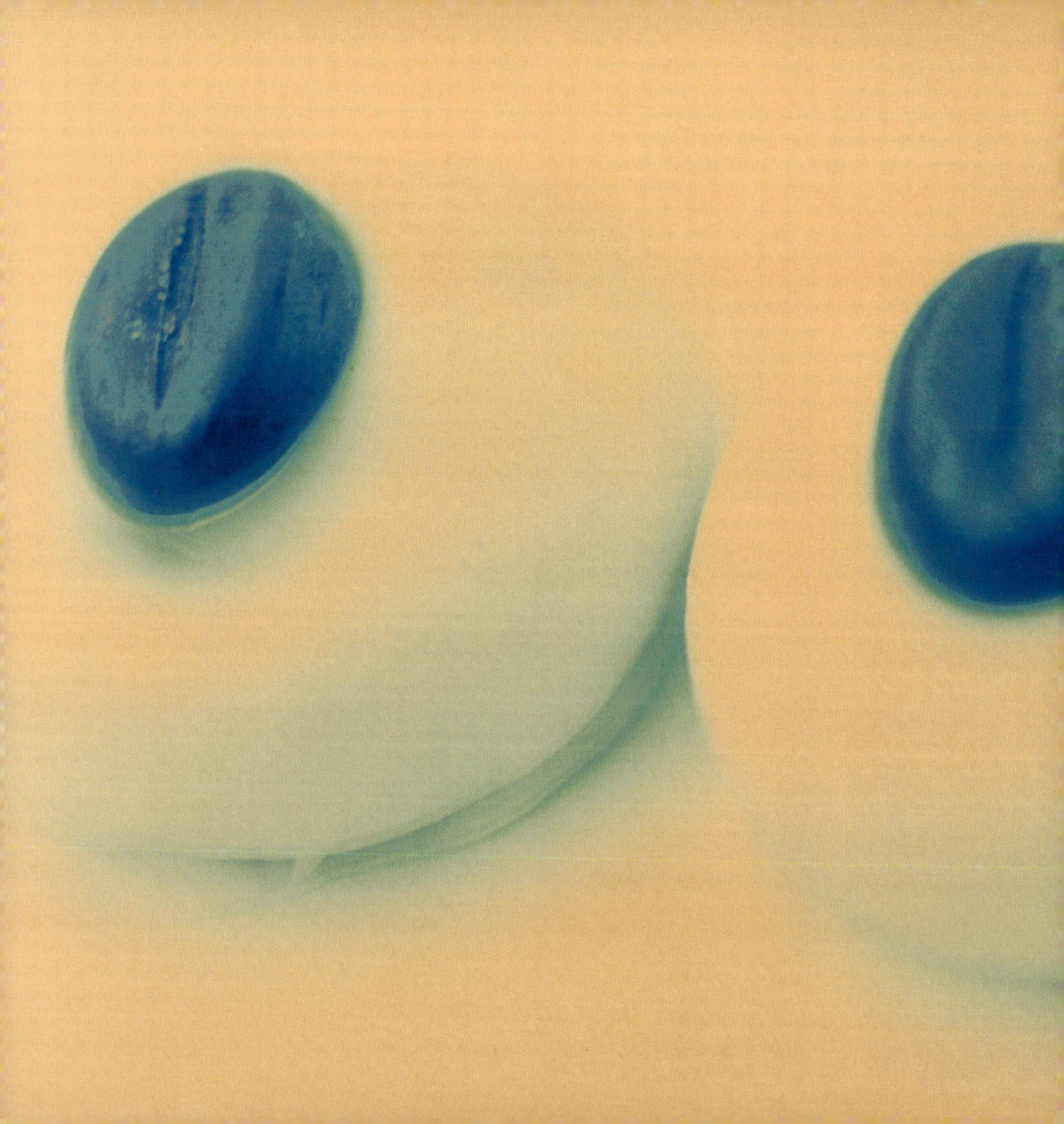

Carrots will not only make your teeth straight, curl your hair and help you see in the dark, they will also add a dash of colour to your sex life. Probably because of the figurative associations of its length and size, the humble carrot was considered an aphrodisiac by the Greeks, the Arabs and throughout the Indian subcontinent. However, the same symbolic characteristics cannot be applied to the onion which, surprisingly, also has an awesome reputation as both a blood purifier and a libido booster.

Artichokes are such a bother to eat, but perseverance should pay off. Not only does the fleshy heart of the artichoke taste deliciously tender, but the vegetable is reputed to cause mild euphoria – and of course peeling off the tips and dipping them in butter or vinaigrette can, in itself, be a very erotic act.

Mushrooms, according to Diana Warburton's *A-Z of Aphrodisia*, are said to be 'redolent of a lover's bed' and to 'smell of sex'. She also maintains that both celery and truffles contain a pig pheromone, which, although it supposedly adds to their licentious reputation, sounds rather strange – unless you are intent on seducing a particular pig. However, history relates that Madame de Pompadour and Casanova were amongst those who used truffles to stoke the fires of passion and, whether you believe in their efficacy or not, truffles are undeniably a highly prized and delicious delicacy.

The young shoots of the asparagus plant, smothered in melted butter and eaten with the fingers, are another ancient food still enjoyed by lovers today, while rocket, so beloved of modern restaurateurs, has been a long-standing ingredient in potions intended to increase ardour. Add it to your salad bowl and the next time you shave a little parmesan on to your mixed leaves, don't forget that dressing is optional.

vegetables

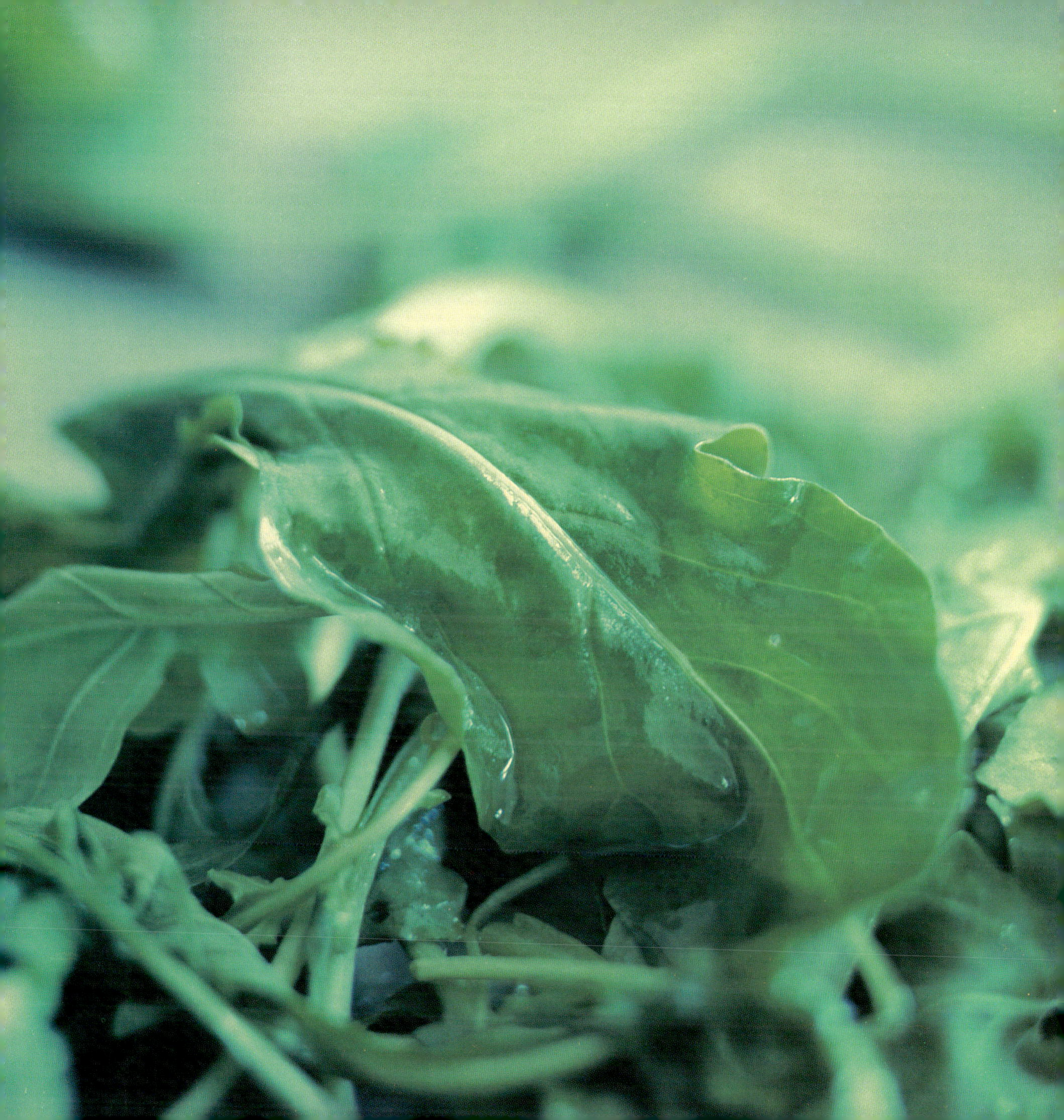

I asked Rosie for her idea of an effective aphrodisiac and she came up with the most popular choice of all: 'Two glasses of wine, preferably champagne.'

Sex without champagne is like taking a bus instead of a chauffeur-driven limousine – you'll get there in the end, but not in anything like the same style. Sex with wine is marginally better, but whether you're travelling in a Jaguar or a Ford Escort will depend on the quality of the wine. There's no doubt that alcohol is a social lubricant and, with its ability to relax and lower inhibitions, it can be a lover's little helper.

Alcohol is the last legal intoxicant. When taken moderately, it certainly increases the libido. However, while it undoubtedly raises the urge to get down and dirty, if you drink too much you will get down and stay down. Alcohol will fill you with desire, but impair your ability to do anything about it. I'm going to gloss over the health considerations here – I'm sure you know it is bad for your liver and your relationship if you use alcohol to excess, but I'm not your mother.

With that in mind, there are an infinite number of cocktails to choose from, some with downright lewd names and even lewder intentions. If you don't fancy those subtle ones like 'a long hard screw', you can opt for a Margarita, a tequila-based drink which allows you to lick salt from the back of your hand in a suggestive way, before downing the liquor.

My friend Sarah takes the simple gin and tonic to new heights of carnal bliss by reporting that just rubbing your hand up and down the smooth sides of your partner's glass can give him an instant erection. I haven't tried it yet, because every time I think of it I see her husband in an entirely new light.

alcohol

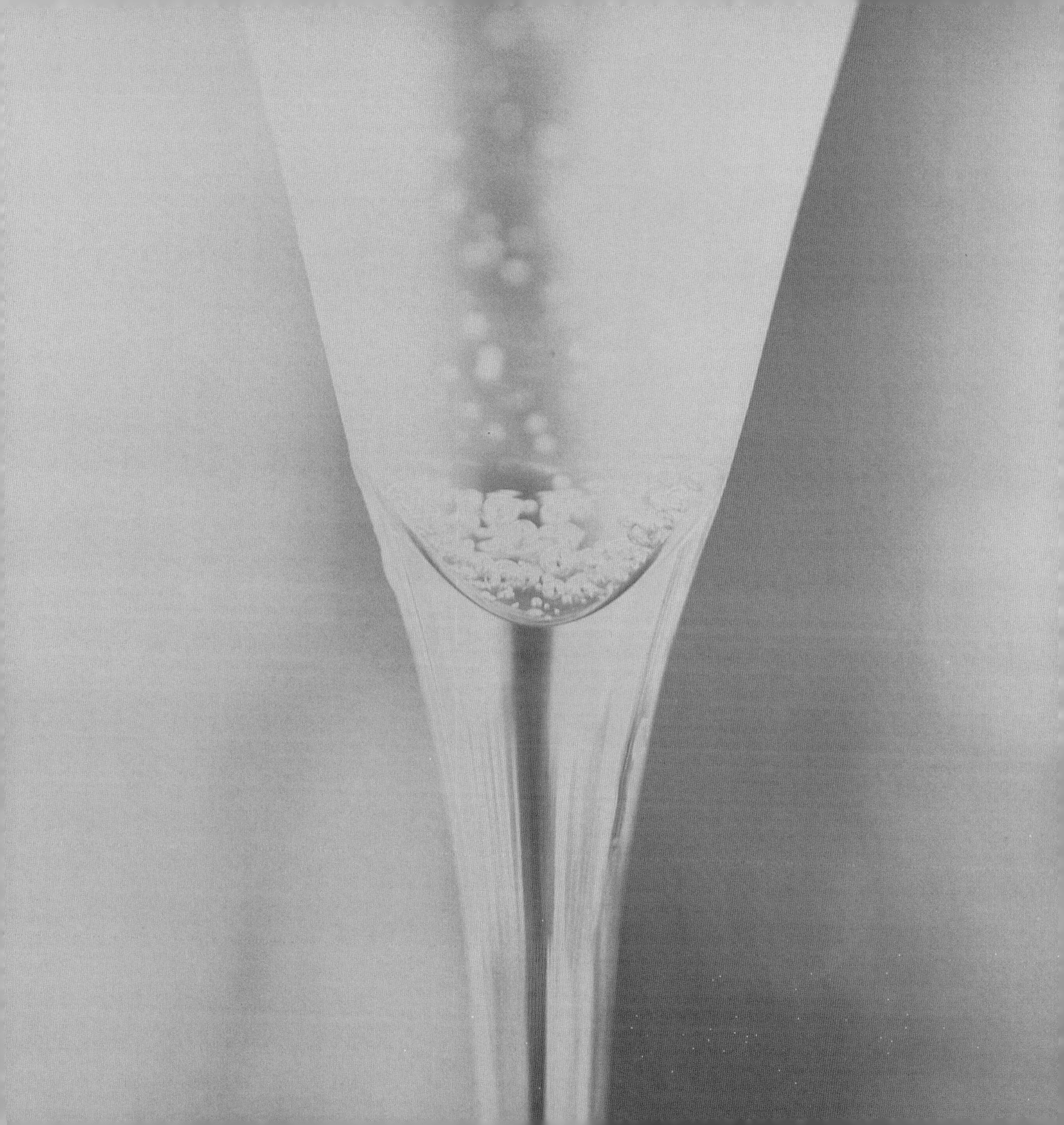

Flowers are not only beautiful and decorative, but also intensely erotic. Artists as diverse as Georgia O'Keefe and Robert Maplethorpe have explored their unashamed sexual imagery in paintings and photographs – it is easy to see why. You have only to look at the most simple flower to see how blatantly erogenous they are.

What makes them so special, however, is not their appearance, but their scent. Imagine sitting outside at dusk when the honeysuckle releases its sweet perfume into the night air or the delicate smell of jasmine drifts through your bedroom window – both scents speak of long, languorous summer evenings when a young woman's fancy turns away from a dozen long-stemmed red roses to other things that happen in the dark.

Smell is said to be one of the most evocative of the senses and can evoke all sorts of half-forgotten memories. I can't smell gardenias without thinking of my honeymoon, and even the clematis scrambling over a garden wall can send me back to a certain event involving an outdoor swimming pool and an American exchange student.

Roses, jasmine, hyacinths, orange blossom, even orchids, have all been endowed with aphrodisiac powers. A room filled with the aroma of flowers may be a perfect setting for seduction, but although those rose petals strewn across the bed might look romantic, they are going to get into all sorts of unwanted places and stick to your body like a second skin. Scatter them instead in a shallow bowl of water with a few floating candles and content yourself with a few drops of rose oil sprinkled on your sheets.

Billie Holiday, the jazz singer, was never without her signature white lily in her hair. However, this was not because of its intoxicating smell, but because she had dozed off while drying her hair and singed it. Now you know what to do if you have a bad hair day. But for men – your partner will forgive the unruly hair quicker if the flowers are cellophane-wrapped instead of stuck behind your ear. Trust me on this one.

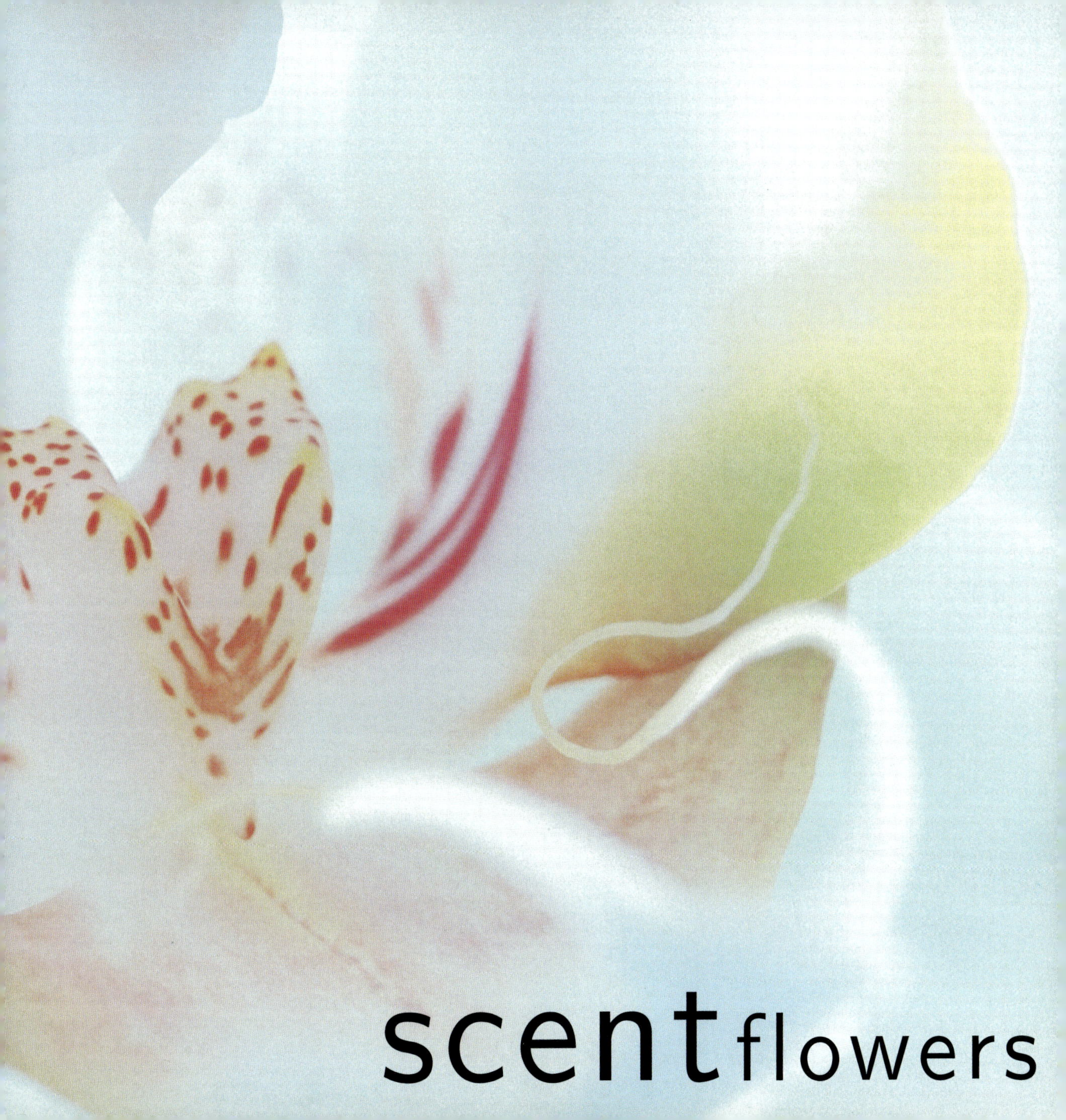

scent flowers

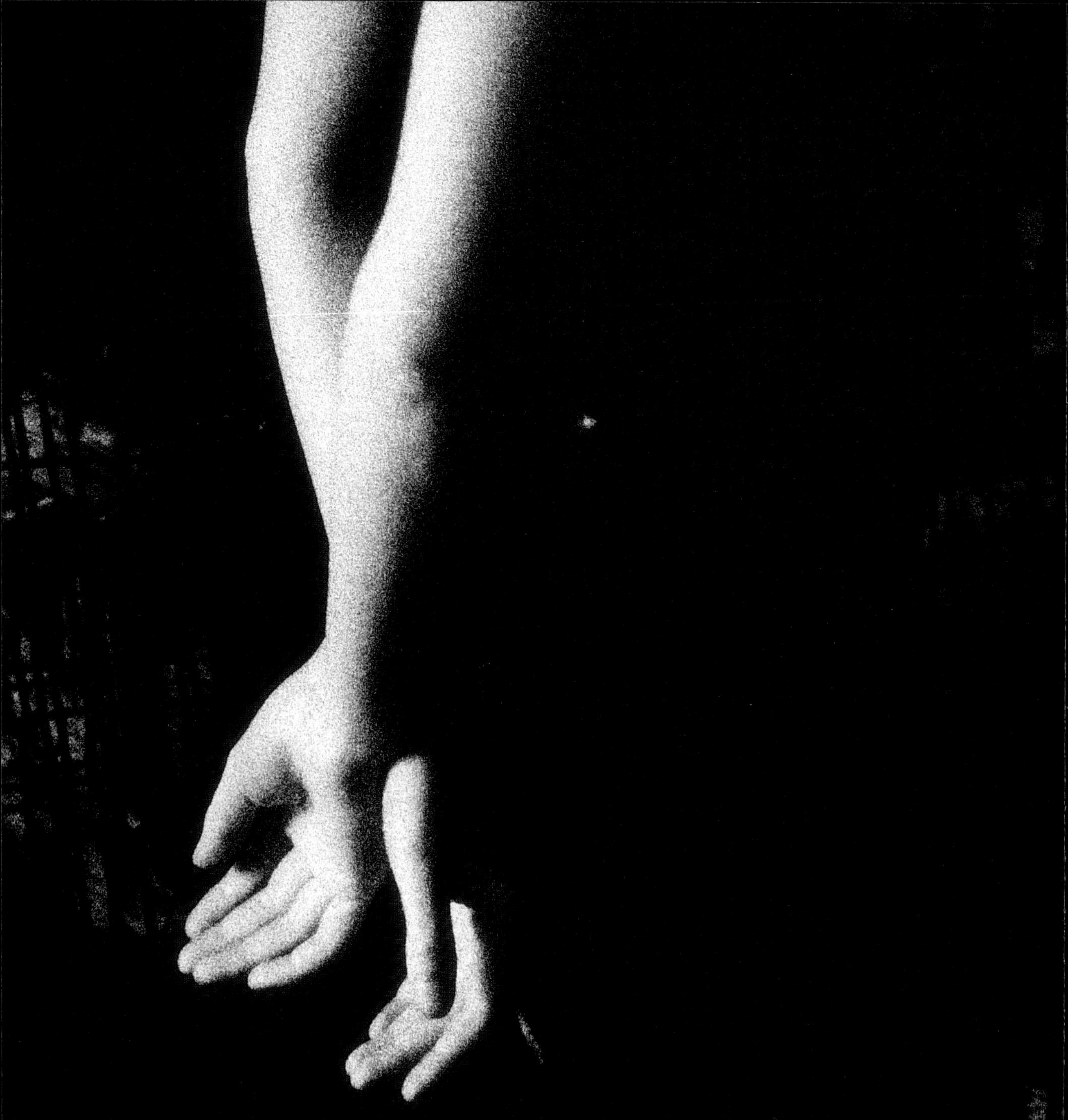

It seems that the periodic table was more than just something you gazed at until the bell rang and the poor, demented chap in the white coat stopped fiddling with his test tubes. Recent studies will make you wish you had paid more attention at school, because scientists have confirmed that there really is chemistry when two people are sexually attracted to each other. Just like animals, we humans give off pheromones which can be detected subliminally by others.

Pheromones are odourless chemicals secreted by animals in order to communicate, amongst other things, sexual desire. Hamsters apparently choose their mates this way – though unless you are particularly fond of hamsters this may not be immediately relevant to your plans for next Friday night. However, even without the severely limited physical criteria of hamsters (let's face it – they do all look the same), a new study has revealed that women also rate how a man smells as one of the prime determining factors in choosing a lover. Sweat, however, did not score highly on the list of sensory stimulants for women, so it's no use waving around that sodden gym vest – it's not going to work.

Obviously, many people do find natural body scents arousing, particularly if the body itself is pleasing to the eye. Pheromones or not, there is nothing you can do for a perspiring Sumo wrestler, but there's a certain animal attraction to be found in a slim-hipped man doing something physical with a power tool.

Of course, they've bottled it. A US company has produced a synthesized pheromone called Athena, which, when mixed with your regular aftershave, has had impressive success in trials. A female version is also available, so perhaps it's time to forget your lucky knickers, girls. Now all you need to find is that construction worker.

pheromones

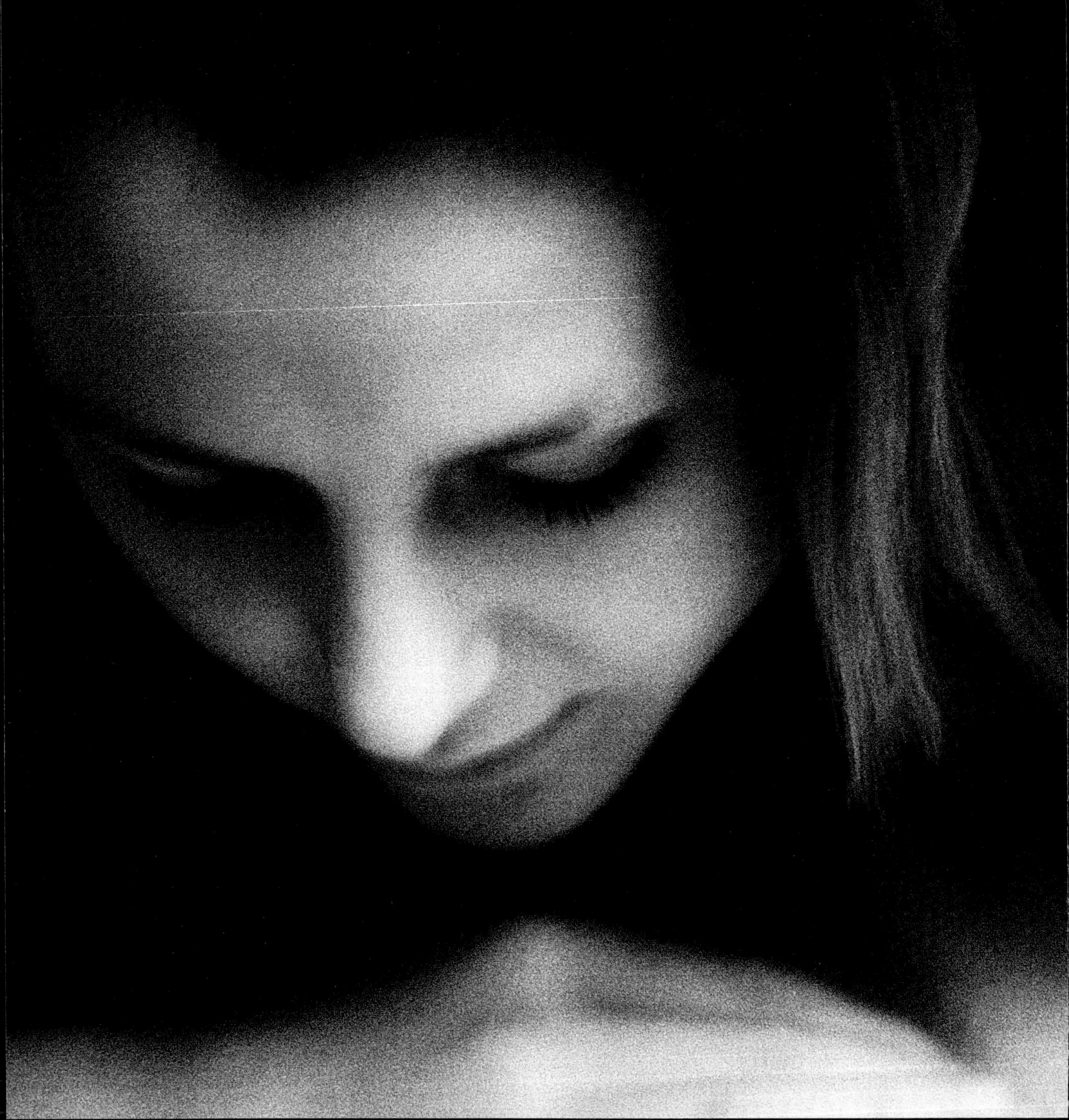

Smell is the Cinderella of the senses, but when you consider that just the faintest aroma can change your mood within seconds, it shouldn't be underestimated. Perfume has been used for centuries to beautify and entrance. Possibly this has been in an attempt to mimic pheromones (see page 61), especially since one of the most popular scents – civet – is said closely to resemble the male sex hormone, testosterone. The perfume industry also uses other animalistic smells such as patchouli and ambergris.

Because smell is the sense that is most closely associated with memory, if you always favour the same perfume then that aroma will become indelibly linked to you in your lover's mind. Weeks later a man might notice another woman wearing your perfume but immediately think of you, even if she is wearing a low-cut dress held up by two tiny straps and a lot of optimism.

Women usually prefer a man to wear more natural or spicy scents, perhaps containing lemon, lime, sandalwood, pine or cinnamon. The important thing with aftershave is to be subtle or you will smell as if you are just off to a gigolos' convention. As a general rule, your cologne should not arrive in the room before you do. If they start publishing your movements in the newspaper next to the pollen count, you are wearing too much.

But no matter how sparingly you apply them, some scents will delight and others repel. Still others will send you sneezing to the bathroom cabinet for an anti-histamine, especially those with a high degree of synthetic fragrances. The purer the scent the better, but experimenting with too many at once will leave you smelling like the inside of a hooker's handbag – so be selective. The only way to be sure that a particular perfume suits you both is to try it out on your partner. If he or she starts opening windows, don't assume it's because of the room temperature.

perfume

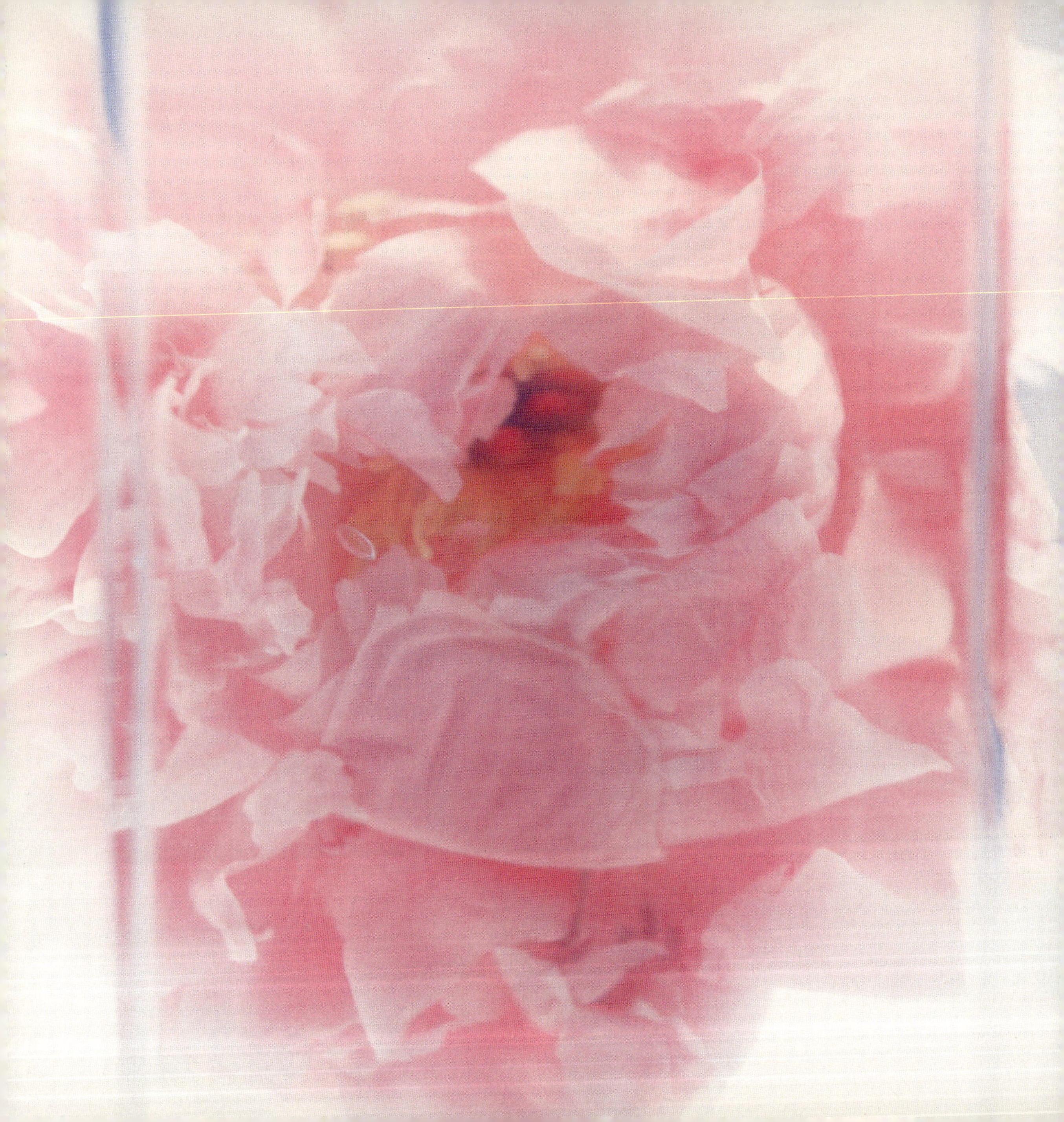

If your love life needs a little rekindling, don't waste time looking for matches – get yourself a few vials of essential oil instead. Aromatherapy is a whole science devoted to essential oils derived from flowers and plants whose effects are both medicinal and mood-enhancing. These oils can be used to the best effect through body massage and inhalation, or by putting a few drops into your bath.

Although you should be cautioned against using certain aromatherapy products while pregnant, essential oils can treat everything from depression to fatigue, as well as encouraging relaxation and well-being. As long as you don't become so relaxed that you fall asleep, they can definitely enhance passion, especially when combined with a sensual massage (see page 39).

Each oil is said to possess its own individual quality. Some are distinctly male in character – like frankincense, myrrh and sandalwood – while neroli, rose maroc and lavender are more female in temperament. Lime and rosemary are both invigorating, lemon is a sedative and even the humble black pepper has the fiery reputation of being hot, vigorous and capable of stimulating the mind. But who really cares about the mind at a time like this?

Ylang ylang might sound like a bad song by the Bay City Rollers, and patchouli oil may remind you too much of flares and tie-dye shirts, first time round, but these oils are both useful for awakening desire. Jasmine, however, is the ultimate aphrodisiac and said to be the sexiest and most seductive essential oil. Unfortunately, it is also supposedly irresistible to cats. If your lover starts to scream out someone else's name at a dramatic point in the evening, check that she isn't yelling at the cat before you put your shirt back on. Unless, of course, your own name happens to be Ginger, in which case you are obviously just being fantastically good in bed.

aromatherapy

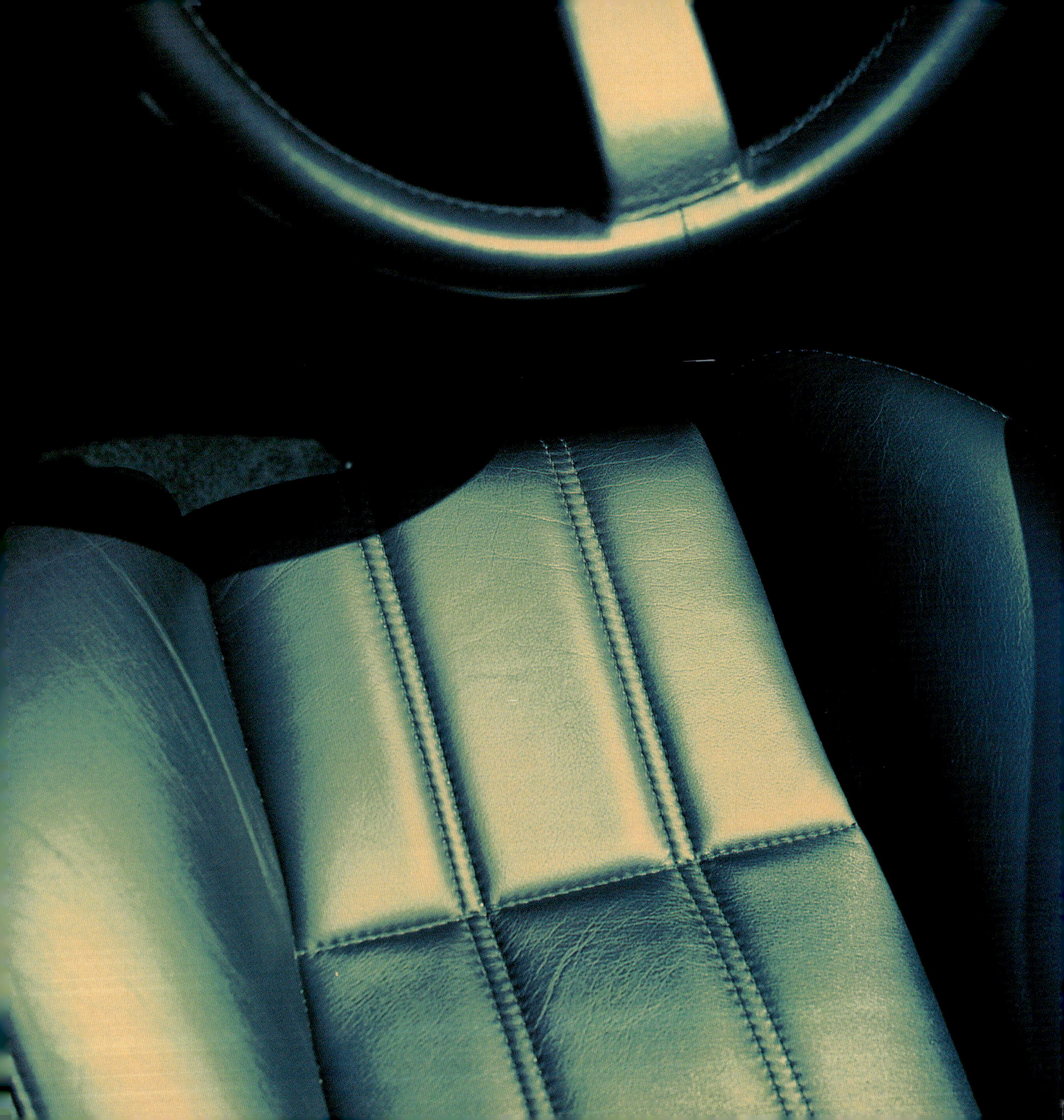

It's uncanny how unscrewing the lid of your sun-tan lotion is like opening a Pandora's box to all those memories of past Mediterranean holidays. Ambre Solaire is like Greece in a bottle; even if you're just rubbing a spot on your legs in the privacy of your own back garden, suddenly there's a strip of white sand, an azure sea and a rather hirsute man called Alexandros.

The smells which unlock your hidden memories can be both varied and strange. For some it's the aroma of cigarette smoke which reminds them, not of the twenty-a-day habit they kicked several years ago, but of a particular night and a particular person. Leather car seats and polished upholstery can make you think of the car your family owned when you were growing up, or the night you lost your virginity in the back of a superannuated Hillman Hunter.

There is no way any potential lover can tap the secret associations which particular aromas have for another. It is also virtually impossible for you to differentiate between a scent that holds a pleasant memory for your partner and one which reminds them of things they'd rather forget. If your lover gives you a certain perfume because he has smelt it on someone else and liked it, pour it down the sink. The someone else could have been his mother, or even his last girlfriend – and these are two parts for which you really don't want to audition.

Better to concentrate on yourself in this instance. If there is a specific smell which intoxicates you, or induces a happy nostalgia, then use it. I like the smell of household scouring cleanser myself, but then I may be just plain peculiar.

scents that stir

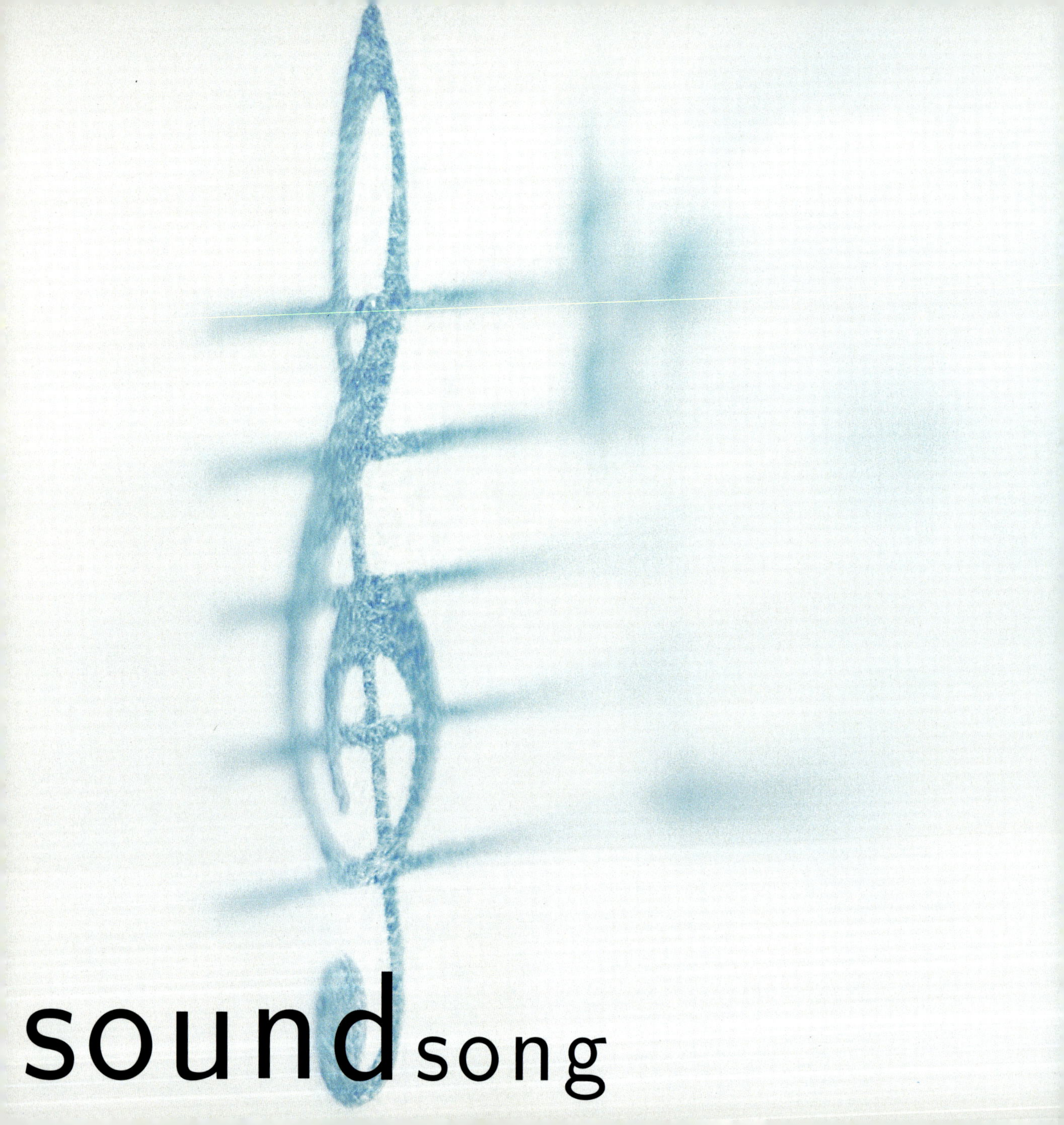
sound song

Ever since the Sirens tried to charm Odysseus with their songs, the human voice has been accorded the power to enchant. Odysseus managed to resist the Sirens' alluring voices by lashing himself to the mast of his boat, but some of us are only too willing to be enslaved by the sound of a beautiful voice.

Unfortunately, not all of us can sing in tune, and if the only siren you resemble is that emanating from a large red vehicle equipped with fire-fighting equipment, it might be best to resort to pre-recorded crooning. Or if, like me, your voice sounds like a heavy chair being drawn across an uneven floor, try singing very quietly and aim for atmosphere rather than applause.

You don't have to possess perfect pitch to seduce with song. It's not just a beguiling melody that puts us in the mood for love, but also the erotic allusions contained in the lyrics. Unfortunately, subtlety doesn't always work – Mary Coughlan, the Irish blues singer, puts it to us straight in her song 'I want to be seduced'. Men should note that, on one occasion when she performed this song live in a club, every single woman in the audience joined in.

However, if music is the food of love, humming is the equivalent of asking the other person at the table to hurry up and finish what they're eating. You will sound bored and deserve to be booed off stage. You should be intent on seduction, not somnolence. And if your partner begins to serenade you, please resist the impulse to sing along with the chorus. You are not aiming to join the Von Trapp Family Singers – you're after a different sort of harmony all together. Think about hitting the high notes and soar.

One of my friends once told me that if any man had ever taken her home and put Leonard Cohen on the CD player, she would have slept with him like a shot. This is where we women are so mystifying to the other sex. Who would imagine for a moment that mournful old angst-ridden Leonard would be a guaranteed turn-on? Most men would have assumed that Leonard Cohen would send a girl screaming for the night bus, not for his magic touch.

But we women are strange, sentimental creatures. We like sad films. We enjoy a good cry. Romance and sad songs go hand in hand – play us some slow, soulful music and whereas a man might be rushing off for a repeat prescription of Prozac by the end of the first five bars, we women will be turning down the lights and getting cosy.

Some music is fornication and nothing else. Mariah Carey or Barry White, the original grunt and groaner, will leave your partner in no doubt that you are in the mood for love, but you'll get no points for subtlety. However, if your lover likes listening to rap, you'll know that a freak is no longer someone who took too much acid in the '60s and that Barry isn't the only one who likes to shoot from the hip.

A man's music of choice might be the theme tune from *Weekend Soccer Highlights*, but even the most hard-boiled man has his romantic side. Try to find out where it is and what records appeal to it before you stun him into submission with *Barry Manilow's Sounds of Seduction*. A blast of loud, pumping rock might be just the thing to drive him wild with lust – as long as it doesn't send him reaching for his air guitar, you are all set for a live performance. Smoochiness is all very well, but a rousing beat can do powerful things to your libido. If nothing else, with the music loud enough to make the room vibrate, you won't be able to do a lot of talking.

music

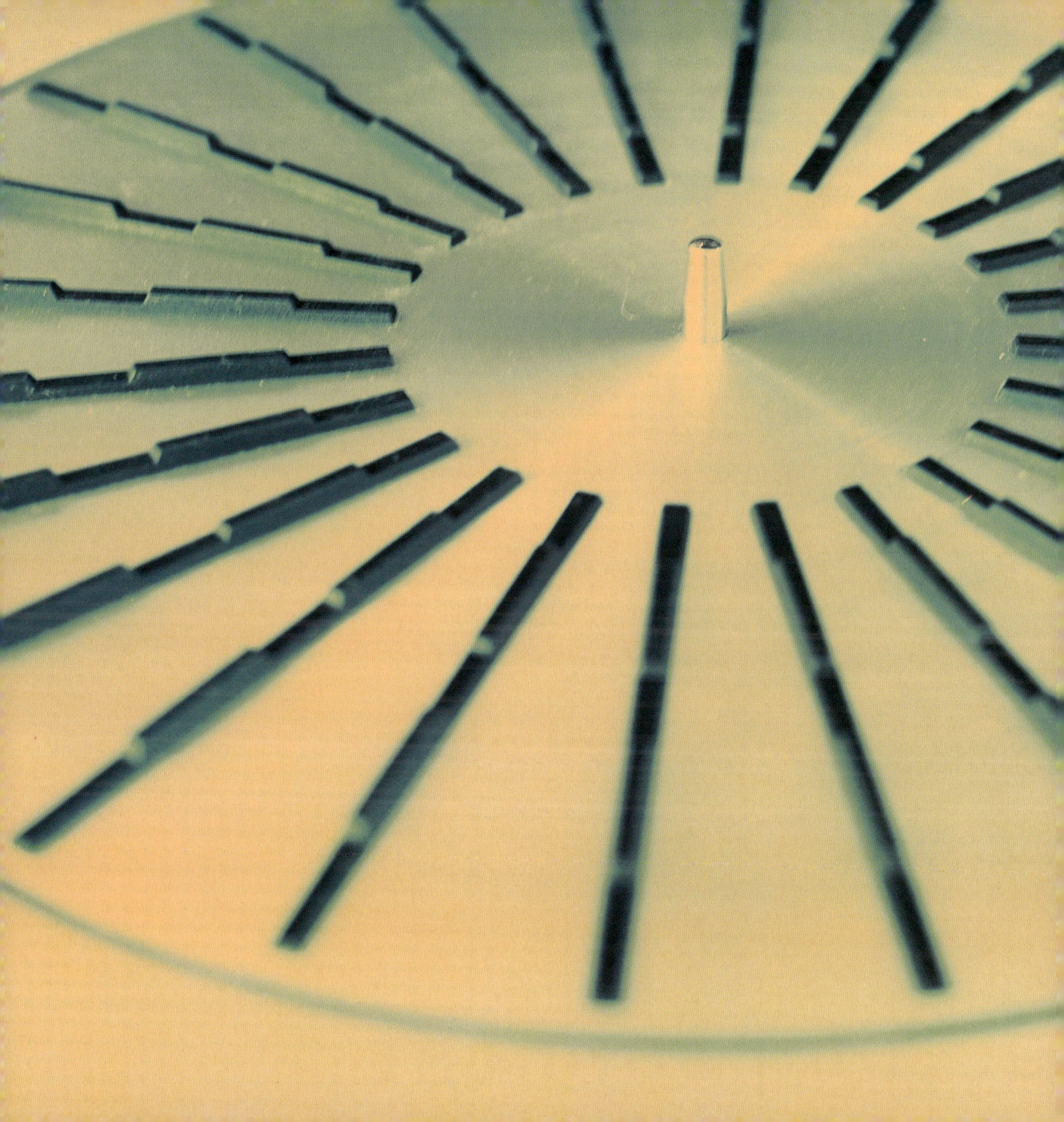

In the film ***10,*** the heroine Bo Derek liked to make love to Ravel's *Bolero*, while in *Sliding Doors* Gwyneth Paltrow came home to find her boyfriend actively engaged in extra-curricular sex to the strains of Elton John. However, outside of the movies, loud music as a background to making love can be more of a distraction than a seduction, especially if your partner starts mouthing along to the words of the song. It is also rather off-putting if the track comes to an end mid-flagrante and your partner asks you to stop what you're doing and change the record. This must be why they have the loop facility on modern CD players.

Most of the women I spoke to said they preferred silence, or at the very least something soft and unobtrusive as an accompaniment. But it's not just sound itself which can be a turn-on; show me a man who knows how to handle a large instrument and I'll show you several moonstruck women. Can there be anything sexier than a man who can draw mellow notes out of a saxophone or a cello, or send shivers up and down your spine just by strumming a few chords on a guitar? Even the oldest and hoariest of blues players can still make their instruments swoop and soar like a passionate woman and fill your mind with lascivious thoughts of surrender. Avoid 'Kumbaya' or anything reminiscent of Saturday night at the youth club, and I guarantee you'll have the woman in the palm of your hand – or anywhere else you want her.

Of course, skill of any kind is awe-inspiring. If that skill is the ability to fill a room with vibrations you can feel from the soles of your feet to the tips of your ears, then it's no wonder rock stars have groupies. It might be no more than a few bars on your clapped-out piano, but any man who can sit down and play it can run his fingers over my keyboard any time.

accompaniment

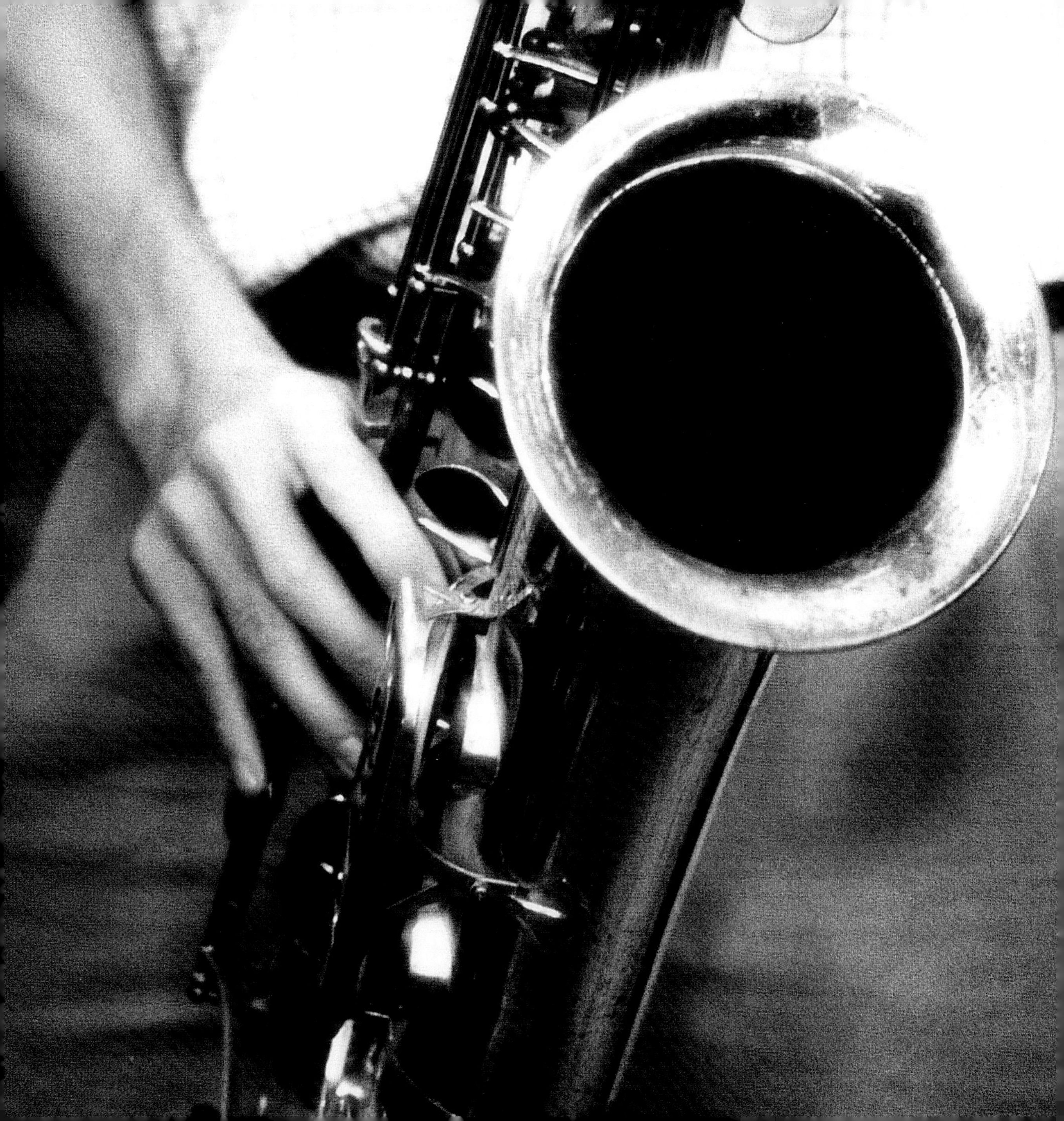

One man's accent is another woman's passport to pleasure. Many of us just love having sweet nothings whispered in our ear, especially if the whisperer has a throaty way of pronouncing his 'r's. A man with an attractive accent has seduction on the tip of his tongue. I once had a French-speaking boyfriend who only had to say my name to reduce me to jelly, even though he always got it wrong. He might, of course, have been confusing me with someone else, but I didn't care as long as he confused me in French.

It's probably not worth taking Linguaphone classes in sex talk for would-be seducers. Easier just to choose a partner from a different country – this gives you an in-built advantage which you should use to the fullest extent. Yes, of course she likes it when, swept away with passion, you start murmuring in Italian. Even better, she doesn't know that you are reciting the contents of your refrigerator rather than spouting off about *l'amore*.

Talking dirty is another conversational gambit that can be exciting to the opposite sex. Personally, I find it doesn't work unless you have a mid-Atlantic accent. 'Do it to me, baby' with a Welsh lilt sounds charming, but vaguely ridiculous if there's supposed to be some kind of inherent earthiness in the phrase.

If you do decide to give your partner a little vocal encouragement, it should sound as if you're cheering him on, in a sensual and generally gratified fashion, rather than giving him a coaching session in your top ten erogenous zones. When I was a student, I once had a bedroom above a screamer who sounded as if she was starring in a B schlock horror movie every time her boyfriend spent the night. I guess he liked it, judging by his smug, love-machine expression. Quiet appreciation, though, does have its advantages – not least that Special Branch doesn't arrive in the middle of the night and stay till breakfast.

accent

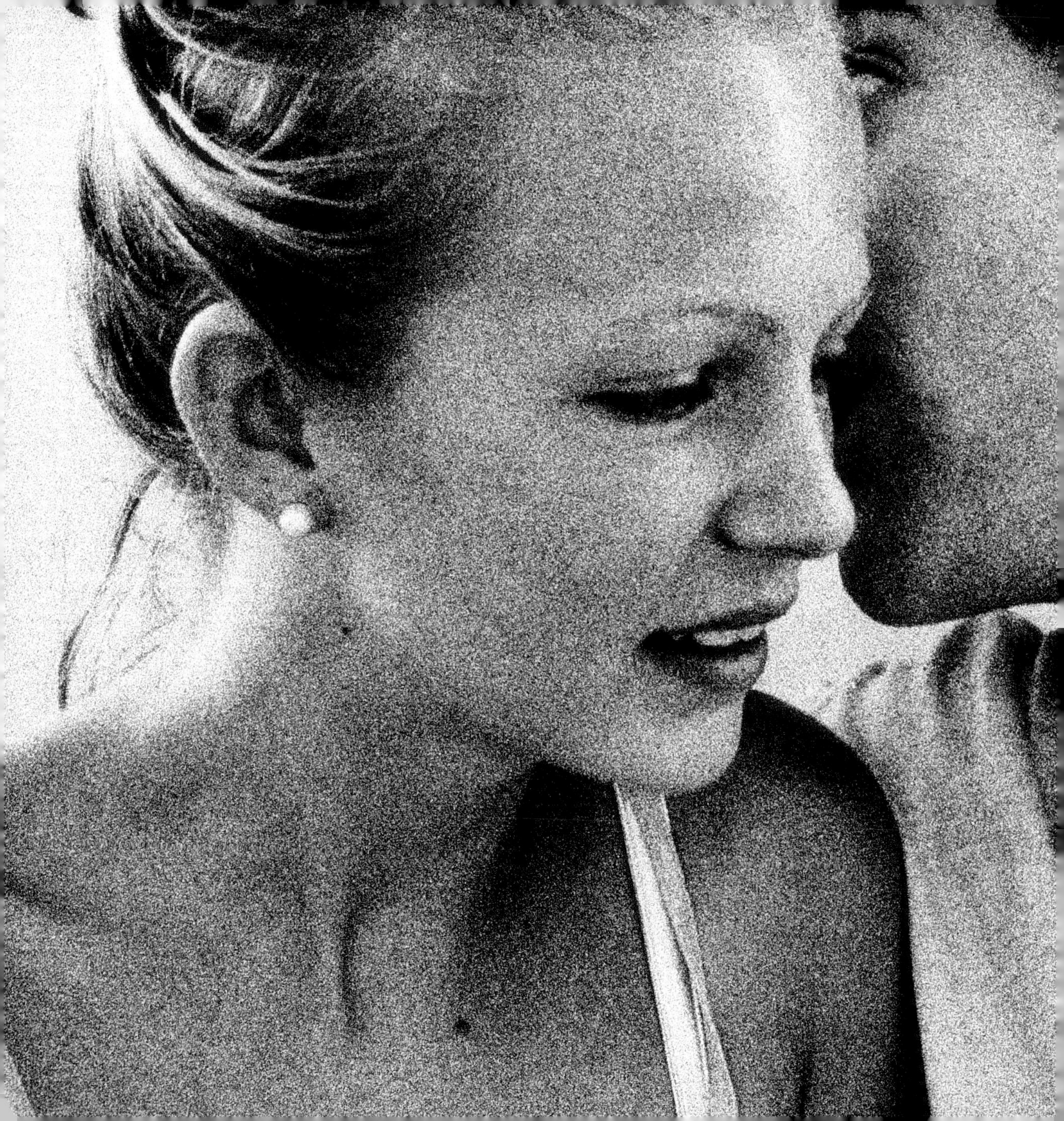

Nature's own soundtrack has the ability to stir our deepest primordial feelings. Who can resist the roar of the surf rolling in against the shore, or the howling of the wind on a stormy night? Rather than acting as a dampener to passion, thunderstorms, accompanied by torrential rain beating against the roof, can instil in us the urge to bolt the door and nestle somewhere warm while we wait until the skies clear.

Elemental sounds such as bird song, waterfalls or the whisper of a gentle breeze often bring with them a feeling of intense contentment and relaxation which can help get you into a sensual frame of mind. You can buy tapes containing everything from Native American chanting to sounds of the rainforest which will transport you and your partner from your studio flat in suburbia to a tropical island beach – well, for 40 minutes or so at least.

A friend says that ever since she saw the scene in the film *Body Heat* where tinkling wind chimes sway seductively during a steamy sex scene, she has found the sound extremely erotic. This explains why her house is festooned with wind chimes – it has nothing to do with feng shui after all. Her husband finds the noise of the wind blowing through a cornfield very sensual because, he claims, it reminds him of the sound made by silk-stockinged thighs rubbing together. It makes me wonder about the nature of their country walks, and just what his wife is wearing underneath the anorak and waterproof hiking trousers.

ambience

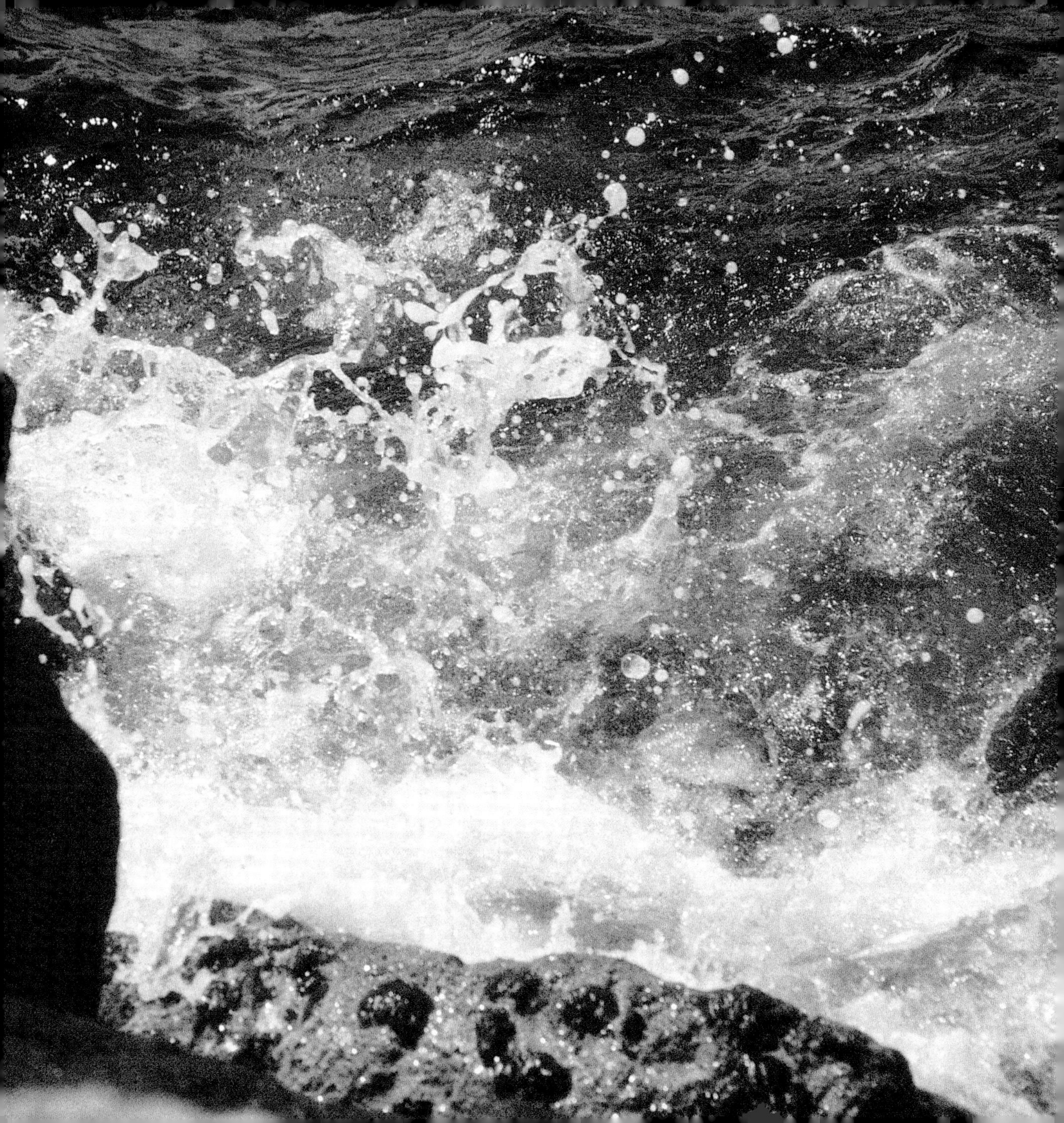

The back row of the cinema is the long-established home of a whole new genre of movies entitled 'Great Films You Kissed Through'. While I won't argue that there are more creative things to do in the cinema than eat popcorn, if you know you won't be keeping your eyes on the screen you might consider renting a few steamy films for home viewing.

This doesn't mean you have wear a wig and dark glasses and go into the back room marked 'Adult Films' – well, not unless your idea of an evening's entertainment is gynaecologically motivated or you are a frustrated linguist trying to broaden your German vocabulary. However, if your partner enjoys this sort of thing – given the anatomical proportions of the actors in such films – you can at least be reassured that he or she doesn't suffer from an inferiority complex.

For the more mainstream viewer there are countless films with very erotic sex scenes, and the added bonus of a coherent plot: *Sea of Love*, *The Big Easy*, *The Postman Always Rings Twice*, *Fatal Attraction*, *9½ Weeks*, *Basic Instinct*, to name but a few.

If you choose anything containing a scene that you'd be embarrassed to watch with your mother, you are on the right lines. Naturally, this excludes videos of you naked in the washing-up bowl at six months old – which are, of course, mortifying, but for different reasons.

If you get to the end of the movie without anyone yelling cut, you can always close the set and have your own instant replay. After all, there's nothing like a live-action film.

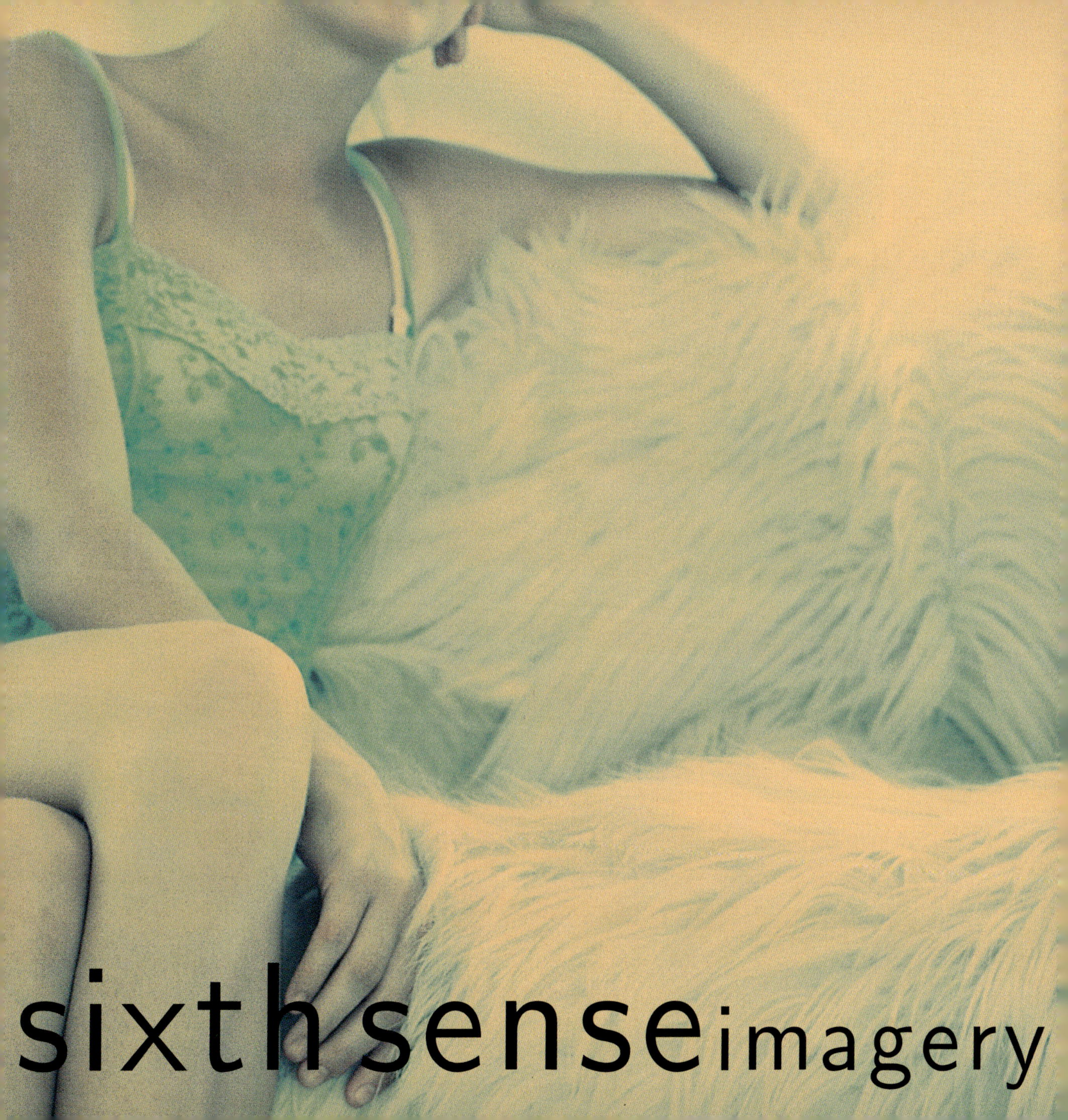
sixth sense imagery

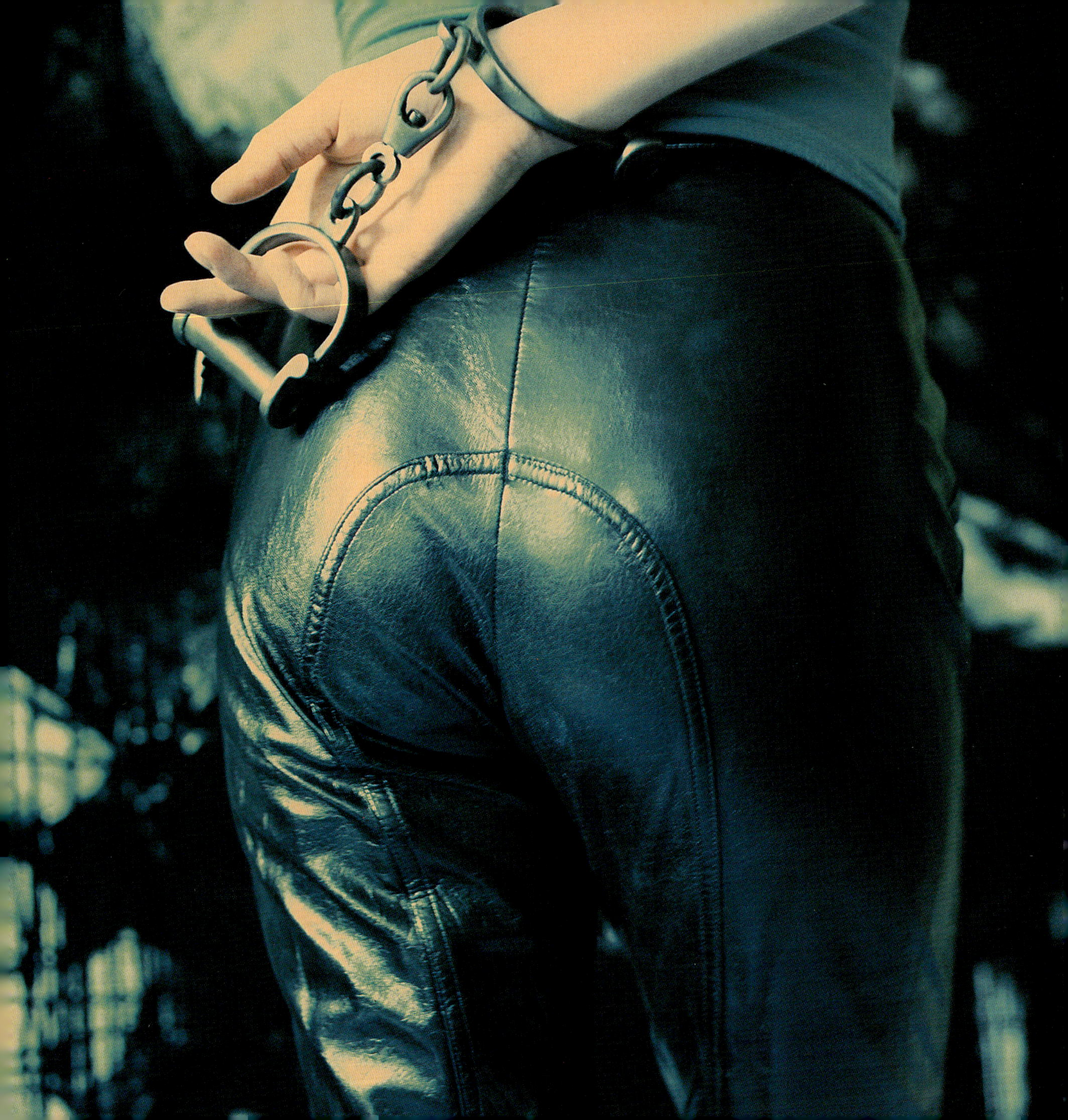

Power is a major turn-on and some women find a man in uniform irresistible. Of course it depends on the uniform – traffic wardens tend to make you fumble for your car keys, not the buttons on your shirt, and security guards are more likely to set off alarm bells than lower your defences. Men may also hunger after authority figures, although often black leather corsets play a larger part in these fantasies than epaulettes and police helmets. When a man arrived to take my cousin out to dinner with a pair of silver handcuffs dangling from the back pocket of his jeans, I wondered if she had known what she was letting herself in for when she answered that personal ad at the back of the *Police Gazette*. It turned out she had.

But power is more than a bit of braid and a row of brass buttons – men in suits who give the impression of being able to juggle foreign currencies whilst curing cancer on their day off often instil us with confidence. This is why they call it power dressing – if he appears self-assured and powerful, then we imagine his expertise extends to other, more sensitive areas.

However, the woman with the sharp suit and an attitude to match can be less of an aphrodisiac to the man who has put his ego down and forgotten where he left it. If he doesn't feel threatened by your red two-piece with embroidered insignia on the lapel, you may have him asking for a packet of peanuts and a double scotch, rather than your telephone number. Thank the great god of padded shoulders that the true potentate is able to cope with the demands of a feisty woman. Still, it might be useful to get that old PVC cat-suit out of storage anyway, just in case you really have to put your foot down.

Hard.

power

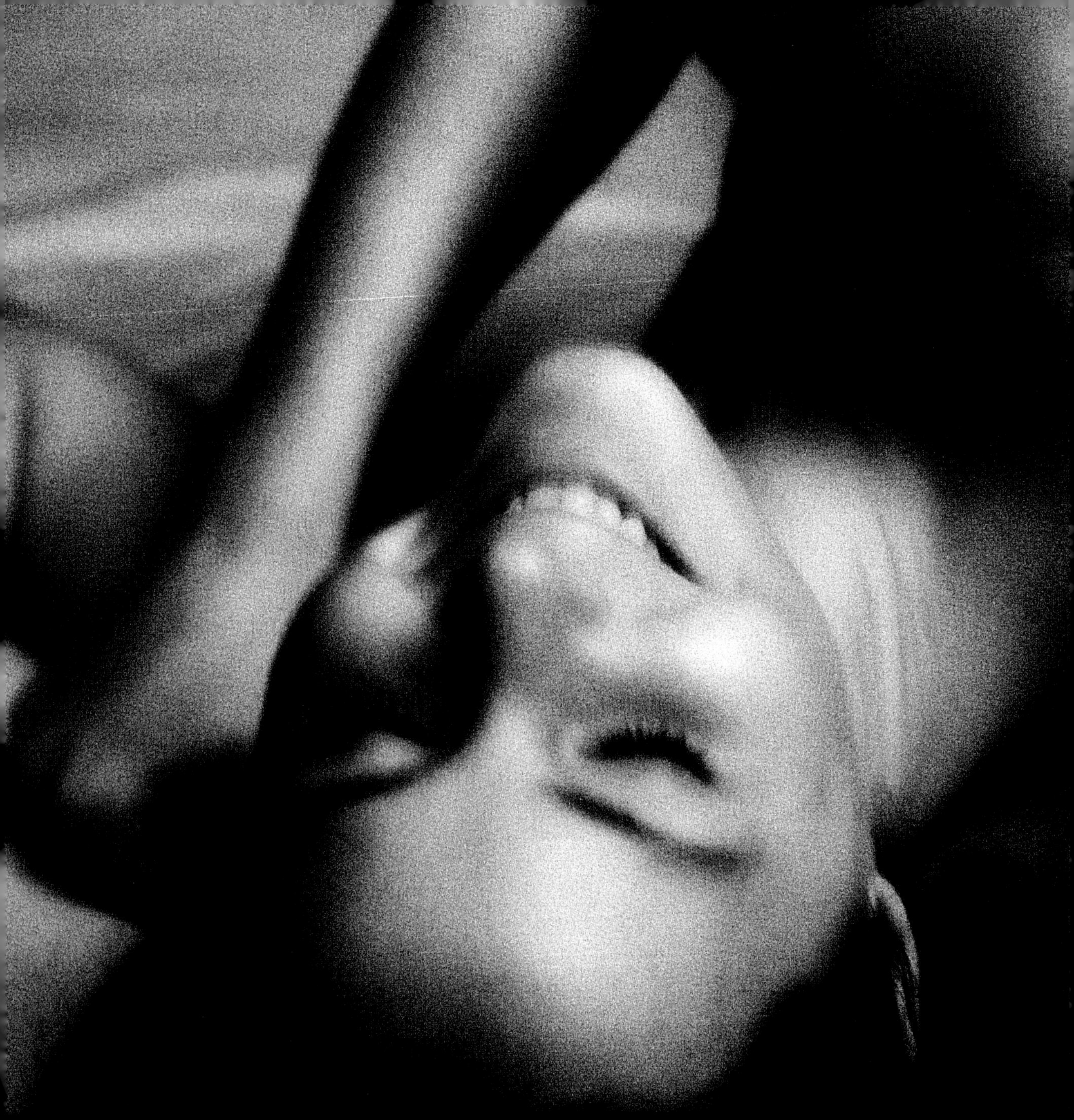

Laughter is supposedly the greatest aphrodisiac of all. However, this does not mean that seduction should involve entertaining your lover with an impromptu performance of your stand-up comedy routine. There are no joke books for swinging lovers. Sit down and forget the buffoonery – you want to stroke the ego, not the funny bone.

Dull people, as well as being chronically boring, often have the added handicap of imagining that others find them amusing. Yawning, no matter what others tell you, is not a sign of hilarity – except perhaps for those lucky people taking the anti-depressant drug Anafranil, which has the unusual side-effect of inducing an orgasm every time you yawn. These people probably love your anecdotes about the day the dog died (oh, how we laughed), but then they probably also love the Home Shopping Network and live in a perpetual state of bored bliss. Just don't give up your day job until you are sure.

We all love a person who can make us laugh, but you don't have to try too hard. It's fine to be amusing, but your lover wants to be charmed by your personality, not tickled by your bird impersonations. Laughter is really about feeling comfortable enough to let go, relax and enjoy yourself. If you share a sense of humour, you will doubtlessly find you can connect in all sorts of other areas.

And if your jokes aren't funny, there's one sure-fire way of keeping you quiet.

laughter

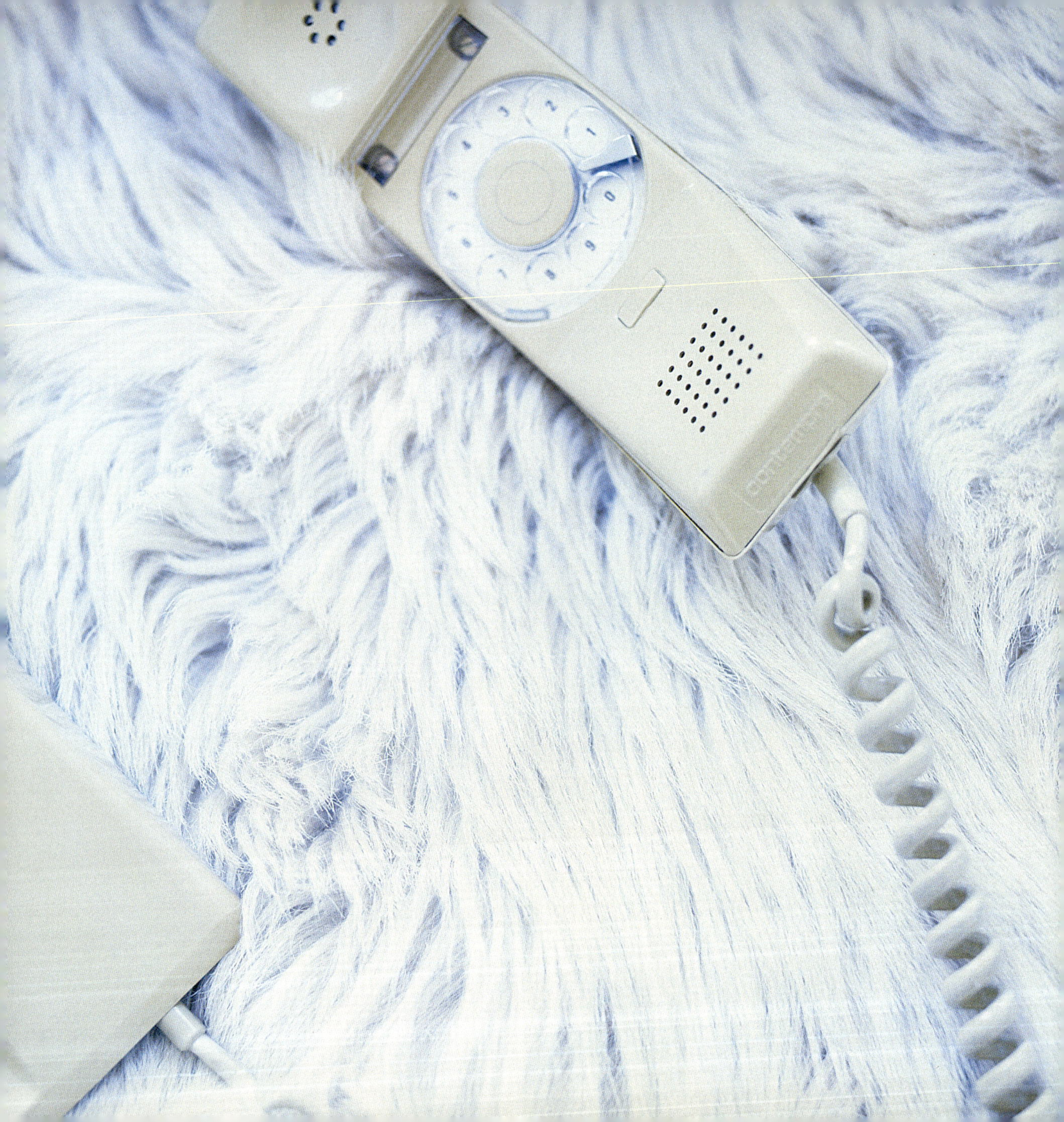

Passion comes in many guises. It can emerge in the way you react strongly in support of a cause, or when expounding a dearly held belief. But it's a shame to waste all that emotion on something that inflames only your temper, when it could be rousing something else altogether. A stimulating argument can expand into other, equally passionate areas of your life.

Some couples enjoy playing power games with each other, but inciting desire with a verbal debate is not the same as arguing – don't wait until things become too heated before you throw in the towel.

At the other end of the spectrum, there's that tingle of anticipation when you and your lover are still not sure of each other. Will he call? Will she be there? That wonderful sense of expectancy mixed with a delicious apprehension about what exactly is going to happen when you next get together.

You can't manufacture it, except perhaps by taking the time to tantalize your partner. Keep him/her guessing and retain some mystery in your relationship. You really don't need to be entirely truthful about your number of sexual partners. Believe me – think of the number and divide it by ten. Brutal honesty is up there with dental floss and men who sleep in their socks as one of the greatest passion killers of all time.

We all like to be appreciated and women especially find it irresistible when a man treats them as if they were quite the most fascinating creature who has ever walked the earth. The fact that this man finds you irresistible is so intoxicatingly erotic that suddenly you think you're Helen of Troy. Do not, repeat not, choose this moment to confide in him about your unique collection of porcelain pussy-cats. Some things you shouldn't even tell your best friend – your stallion might turn out to be a mere Trojan horse, and bolt.

conflict

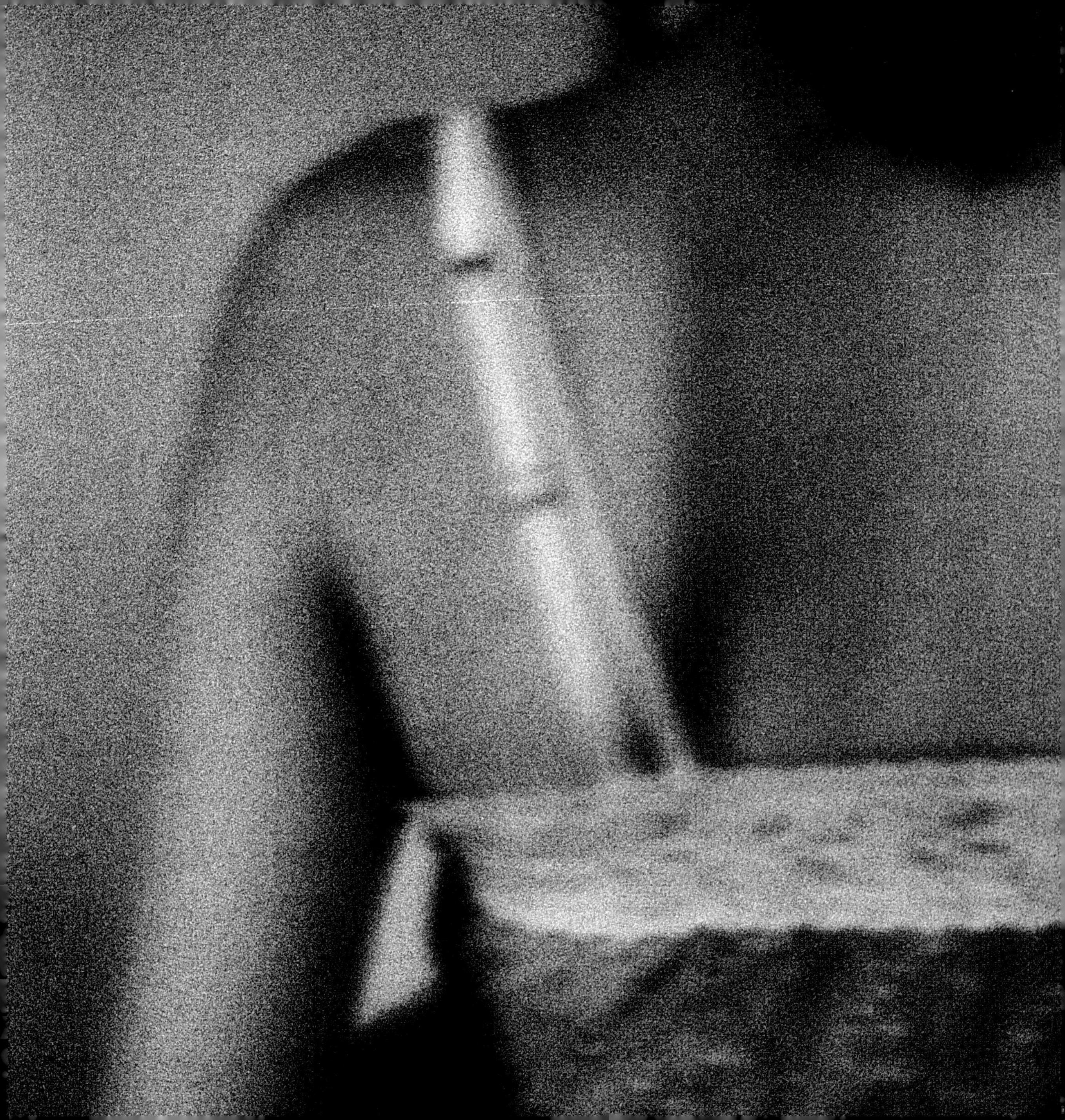

One of the best ways to breathe fire into a relationship which is merely smouldering when it should be raging out of control is the tried and tested dirty weekend. Isn't this what country hotels are for? Surely no one goes to the country for long nature walks? A successful dirty weekend is one in which the great outdoors remains virginally untouched while you practise your orienteering skills between the sheets.

Hotels were invented for two things – sex and room service. Breakfast in bed, lunch in bed, supper in bed – the only thing that should leave the room is the do not disturb sign. Pack a toothbrush and a blindfold for all those games you can only play in the dark. Fill the jacuzzi with bubbles, take your own champagne and send out for ice.

For those who prefer the buzz of city life, all you need is a credit card. New York, Paris, Venice – every major city in the world has numerous discreetly decadent places designed exclusively for love in the afternoon. One London hotel, a favourite for lecherous liaisons, has several exotic bedrooms – there are four-posters, round beds, Moroccan rooms and even one suite with a sunken bath and an open fire. A certain rock star is reputed to have kept his pet python in the bath there. Generally, however, if take your lover away for the weekend, it's better to leave your pets at home. Props are fine – but something warm-blooded usually helps.

Some friends rented the house where the film *Sense and Sensibility* was shot. The location alone was enough to transpose their normally unassuming partners into tall Regency men clad in riding breeches and shiny black boots, while the women swooned, clutched their breasts and murmured, 'Oh, Mr Willoughby.' No one could sleep for the noise of bodices ripping.

But don't worry – it's perfectly acceptable to come back from a lovers' weekend with sleep deprivation and sensory overload. Only unemployed actors rest.

escape

Imagination is a key which can unlock all your secret desires. You have only to look at any book by Nancy Friday to see that people of both sexes have weird and wonderful fantasy lives. And if you decide to explore some of your own daydreams, there is limitless scope for experimentation.

Similarly, fiction – even the literate kind without full colour pictures of pneumatic women – can send your imagination racing off into hitherto dark, forbidden realms. Whenever I go into a bookshop I am struck by how many people seem to be hanging around the shelves containing erotica. Sexually explicit fiction, together with cookery books and self-help manuals, seem to satisfy the entire reading public. So if you are hoping to meet a wildly libidinous cook who is in touch with his inner child, there are worse places to start than your local bookshop. At the very least you'll find a couple of nice recipes, enhanced mental health and a sizzling good read.

But some fantasies lose their power when you vocalize them. As with favourite shirts, after months of use you suddenly grow tired of them and have to switch to something else. A friend talks about 'dusting down' her fantasies from time to time to keep them fresh, and since they seem to include half the men she meets, she is obviously not short of material.

Everyone needs a similar flexibility in their love life. A good lover should be imaginative and innovative, and while this doesn't mean you have to be a graduate of the School of Carnal Knowledge, it doesn't do any harm to enrol for a term or two. However, the marvellous thing about using your imagination is that even if your lover has poor handling and thinks the G spot is an optional extra on a four-door family saloon, when you exercise the power of thought, you can drive your own car. Anywhere you want to go.

imagination

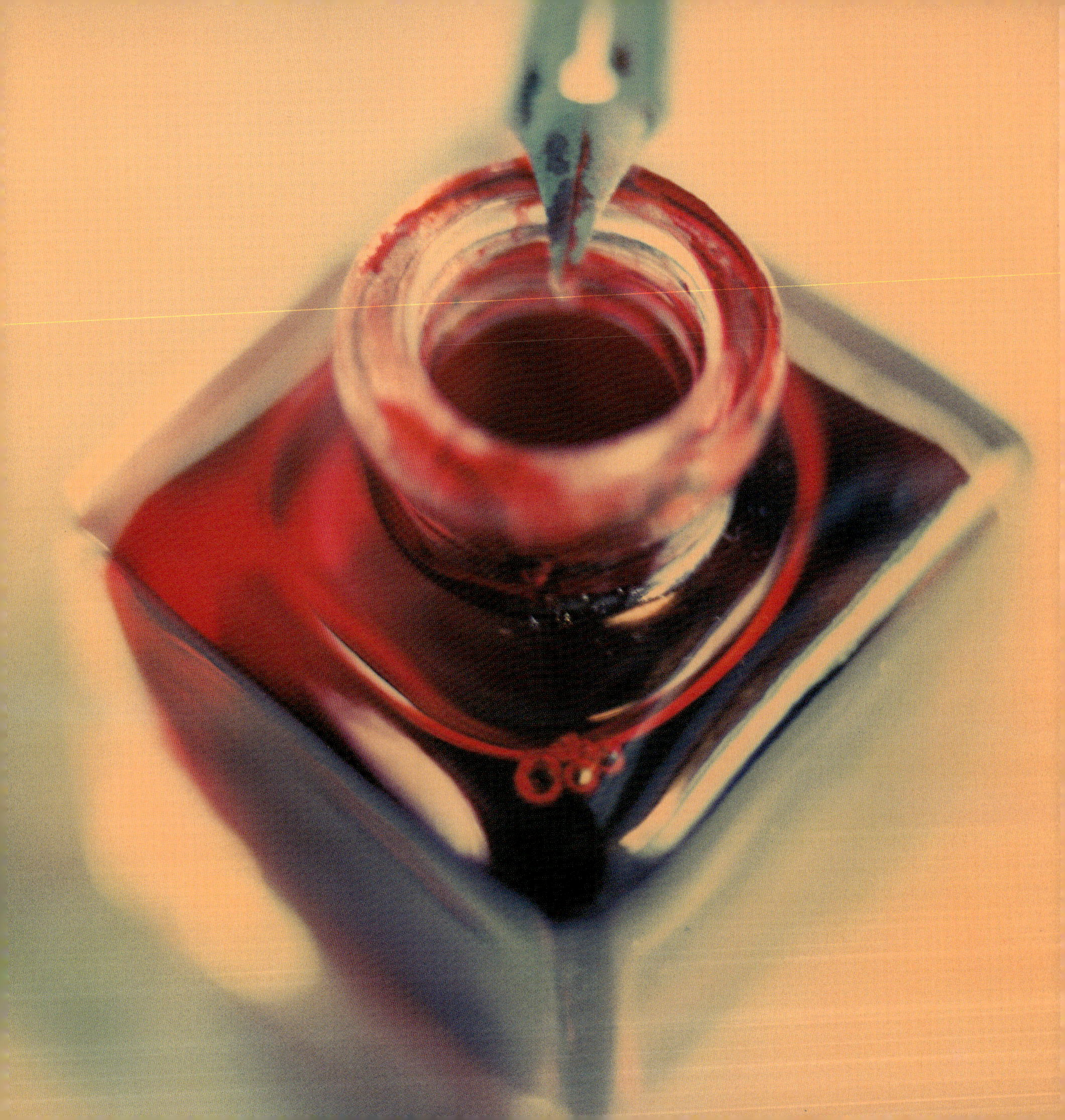

Since the earliest times, lovers have been unable to resist putting pen to paper. From the Bible onwards, poets and writers have celebrated the physical love between a man and a woman with words.

Fortunately, the tradition of love poetry continues today. Those of us without the gift of rhyming couplets can always buy a book of poetry and have that gift-wrapped instead. It's much better to underline a phrase or two of good verse than to write something that sounds as if it comes from the inside of a greeting card. If you're not sure whether or not you've renewed your poetic licence, content yourself with a few lines on a florist's card, and send roses.

If verse fails you, there's always the ancient art of letter writing. The world's great lovers have all conducted voluminous erotic correspondences, and as long as you can manage to string three coherent words together, own a dictionary and don't write in capital letters, there's nothing to prevent you trying a literary seduction yourself. But, although it is possible to be enticed by erotic prose and sizzling innuendo, if you think punctuation is something that happens to tyres, maybe you should just leave a sultry message on the answerphone instead.

Thankfully for the grammatically challenged amongst us, modern technology is on our side. Anyone with a modem and an e-mail address can get on-line and indulge in a virtual romance. With e-mail's informality, you don't even need to use your real name, let alone a capital letter.

Hardly anyone I know has escaped the e-mail affair. Finding an illicit message waiting for you in the electronic ether turns typing into a form of very intimate, erotic foreplay. However, given the anonymity of the Internet, you may never know whether the 36-year-old silver-tongued flautist from Manhattan being 'virtually' seduced by your words is really a man with six chins and a job bagging groceries. Cellulite may not exist in cyberspace, but there comes a time when you have to brave the world and say, 'To hell with virtual reality – let's have lunch.'

printed passion

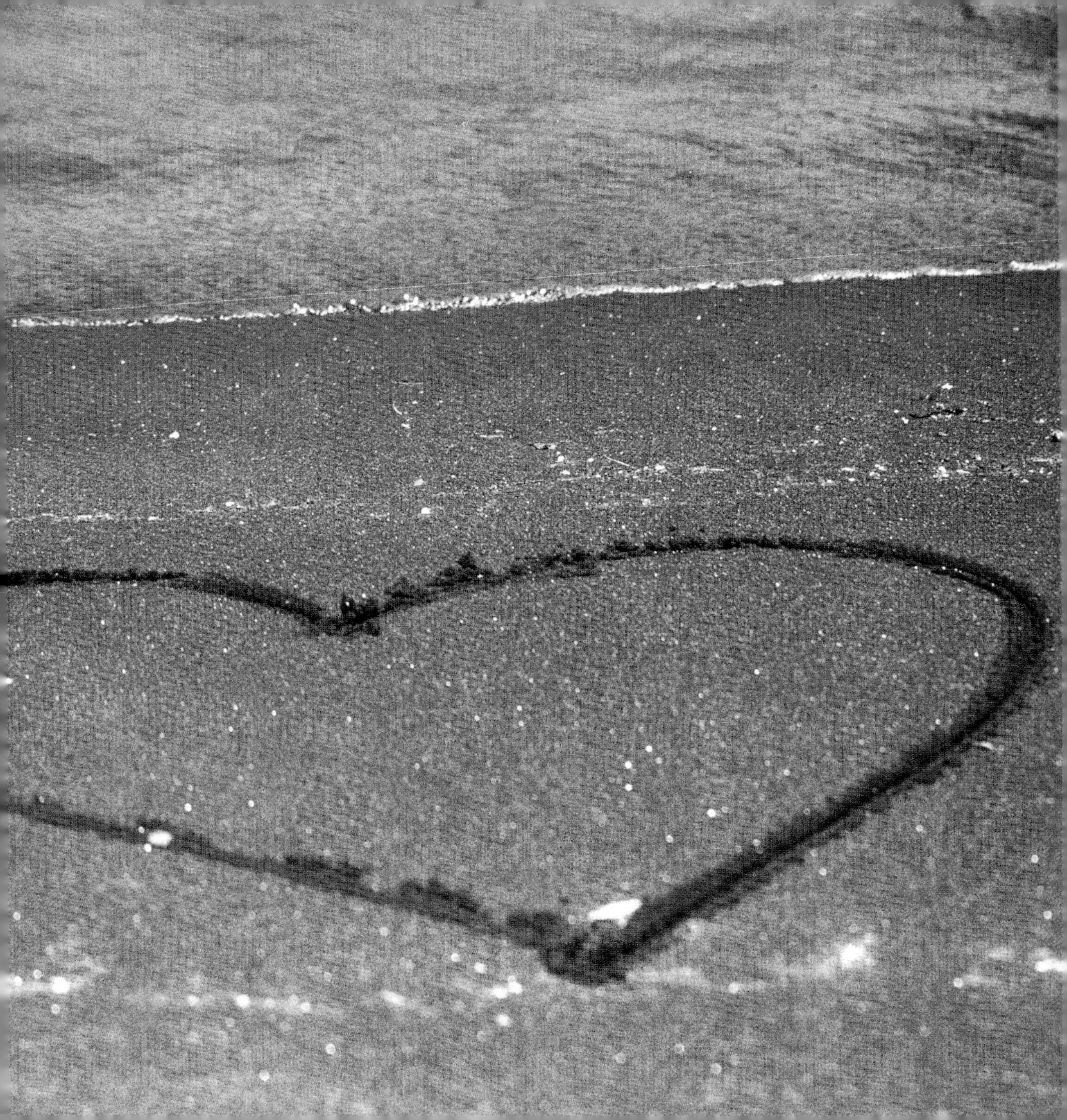

The exhilarating thrill of romance is without doubt one of the most consistent and enduring aphrodisiacs of all. However, romance itself is difficult to sustain, and unless you are committed to a life consisting only of serial relationships, sooner or later some of the novelty is going to fade from even the most ardent affair.

Familiarity can often breed contentment, and contentment, while being comfortable and secure, is not always sexy. Ten years into even the best relationship you may find that the only thing that makes your heart pound is too much caffeine. This is nothing to do with love, or the lack of it – but when you put your libido away in a safe place, it's all too easy to forget you still have one.

Every passionate encounter requires a frisson of mutual attraction, a degree of uncertainty and a jolt of sexual electricity. Long-term lovers need to find a way to short-circuit the procedure and inject a power surge of excitement into their sex life. Think of the passion you felt for your partner when you first met. Remember the fun of flirting. The thudding heartbeat, the breathless moment when you first touched, the sudden lightness in your chest, like being whisked upwards on a fairground ride. Of course, one of the delights of a familiar lover is that when it comes to foreplay, they don't waste time loitering on planet vague. They know exactly where to begin the countdown to blast off. However, sex without a map can be fun. Sometimes it's good to take a detour and get lost again. Either that or redecorate the bedroom ceiling.

Steady relationships don't need to be staid. If you have settled down in Dullsville, you both need to get the hell out of town, fast. I know the Beatles said 'All you need is love', but they forgot the most important thing of all. You need lust.

Buckets of it.

romance

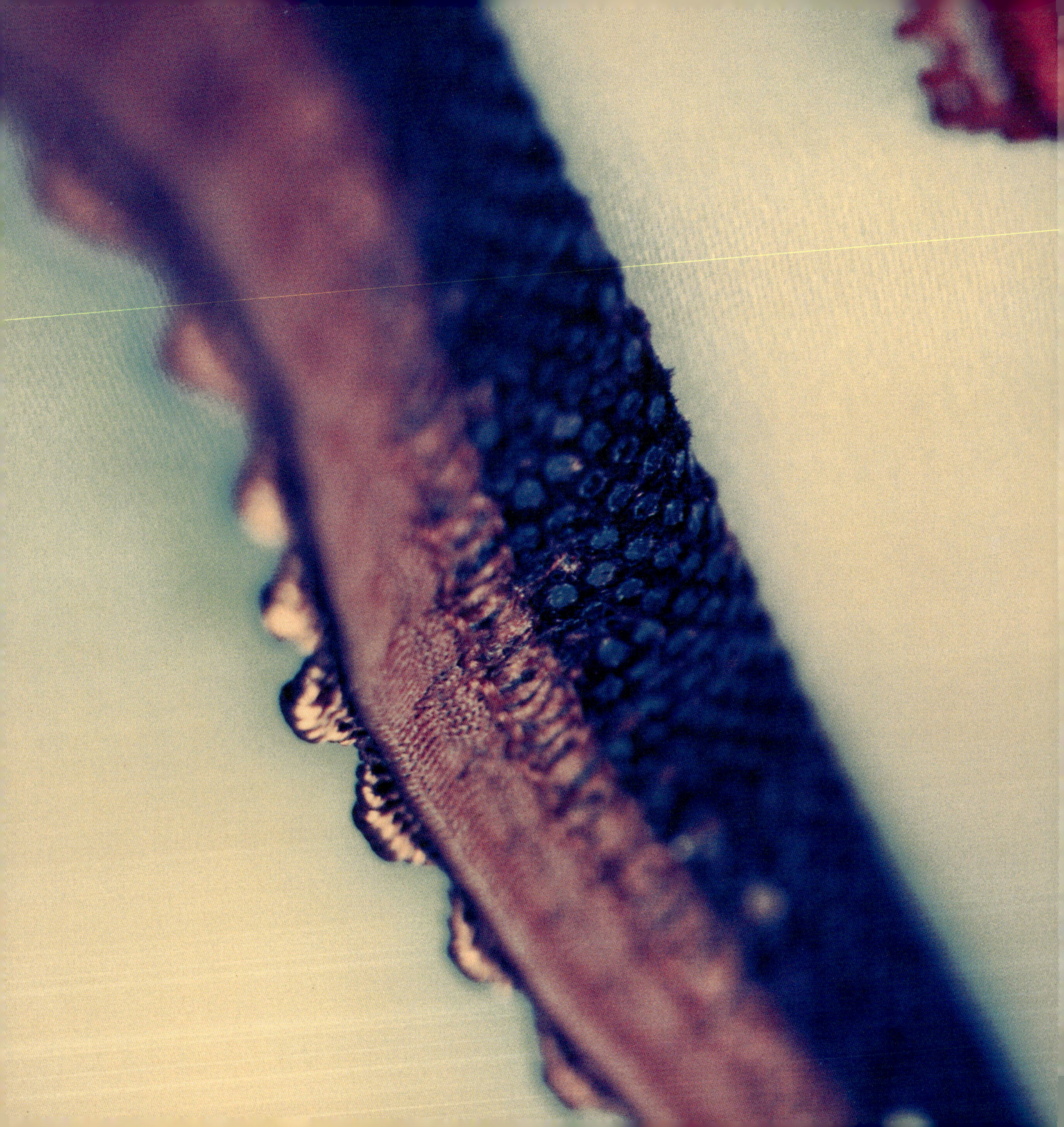